On Fluoridation of Chewing Sticks (Miswaks) with Respect to Dental Caries

Hosam Baeshen

Department of Cariology
Institute of Odontology at Sahlgrenska Academy
University of Gothenburg, Sweden

UNIVERSITY OF GOTHENBURG

وزارة التعليم العالي
Ministry of Higher Education

MINISTRY OF HIGHER EDUCATION SAUDI ARABIA

Gothenburg 2010

Abstract

On Fluoridation of Chewing Sticks (Miswaks) with Respect to Dental Caries

Hosam Baeshen, Department of Cariology, Institute of Odontology, Sahlgrenska Academy, University of Gothenburg, Box 450, SE-405 30 Gothenburg, Sweden

The chewing stick known as a "Miswak" is a natural toothbrush that is widely used for cleaning the teeth. It has been used for thousands of years in Asia, Africa and the Middle East. The aim of this thesis was to evaluate the Miswak as a vehicle for fluoride delivery in the oral cavity. *In vitro* studies showed that both fresh and old Miswaks take up fluoride, which can even reach the pulp of the stick. *In vivo*, the fluoride release from Miswaks impregnated in 0.5% NaF was rapid and was estimated to be around 0.4 mg. A large variation in fluoride release was observed between Miswaks purchased from different stores. This variation may depend on differences in wood properties or the fact that some stores sell fresh Miswaks, while others sell older types. Based on *in vivo* data, it is recommended to use fresh Miswaks impregnated in 0.1% NaF or a maximum of 0.5% NaF on daily basis. The mean salivary fluoride concentration for Miswaks impregnated in 0.1-0.3% NaF produced about the same fluoride level in saliva as toothpaste containing 0.32% NaF.

The fluoride concentrations at the various sites in the oral cavity were higher before than after debonding in orthodontic patients. Moreover, products with a high fluoride content (toothpaste, solution and Miswaks) resulted in higher fluoride retention than the corresponding products with a lower fluoride content. In whole saliva, the highest area under the curve (AUC) values were found in patients using 0.2% NaF rinsing solution, followed by 1.1% NaF toothpaste ($p < 0.05$). The mean fluoride concentration in approximal saliva was higher for Miswaks impregnated in 0.5% NaF compared with other fluoridated products ($p < 0.001$). Consequently, presence of fixed orthodontic appliances appears to increase the oral fluoride retention for all the tested home-care fluoride products.

The treatment effect of fluoridated Miswaks was evaluated on white spot lesions (WSL) in healthy adolescents with a minimum of 4 WSL after completing the orthodontic treatment. They participated in a double-blind, randomised, longitudinal trial, lasting for 6 weeks, and were divided into two groups using: 1) fluoridated Miswaks impregnated in 0.5% NaF (test group, n=19) and 2) non-fluoridated Miswaks (control group, n=18). A custom-made mouth tray, covering half the dentition in the upper jaw, was used while brushing with the Miswaks 5 times/day. The lesions were scored at baseline and 2, 4 and 6 weeks after debonding. The DIAGNOdent readings and the International Caries Detection and Assessment System (ICDAS II) index of the WSL decreased in the test group on the uncovered side of the dentition but not on the covered side, during the 6-week trial ($p < 0.0001$). This indicates that the frequent use of fluoridated Miswaks had a remineralising effect on WSL.

In conclusion, NaF-impregnated Miswaks produced a rapid release of fluoride *in vitro*, as well as *in vivo*, and may be an interesting vehicle for home-care use for caries prevention in countries where they are frequently used.

Key words: Approximal area, caries lesions, chewing stick (Miswak), fluoride, fluoride retention, fluoride solution, fluoride toothpaste, impregnation, orthodontic patients, saliva, Salvadora Persica

ISBN 978-91-628-8039-2
Correspondence to: drbaeshen@me.com

Contents

Papers I-IV

Original papers

This thesis is based on the following four papers, which will be referred to in the text by their Roman numerals:

I. Baeshen H, Kjellberg H, Lingström P, Birkhed D. Uptake and release of fluoride from fluoride-impregnated chewing sticks (Miswaks) in vitro and in vivo. Caries Res 2008;42:363–368.

II. Baeshen H, Birkhed D. Release of fluoride from fresh and old fluoride-impregnated chewing sticks (Miswaks) in vitro and oral retention in vivo. Oral Health Prev Dent;2010;1:93-99.

III. Baeshen H, Kjellberg H, Birkhed D. Oral fluoride retention in orthodontic patients with and without fixed appliances after using different fluoridated home-care products. Acta Odontol Scand 2010, in press.

IV. Baeshen H, Lingström P, Birkhed D. Effect of fluoridated Miswaks (chewing sticks) on white spot lesions in post-orthodontic patients evaluated by DIAGNOdent pen and ICDAS II. Am J Orthod Dentofacial Orthop 2010, accepted.

Introduction

Dental caries is the localised destruction of susceptible dental hard tissues by acidic by-products from the bacterial fermentation of dietary carbohydrates [Marsh, 1999; Marsh et al., 2003; Fejerskov et al., 2003]. The disease process is initiated within the bacterial biofilm (dental plaque) that covers a tooth surface. The very early changes of caries in the enamel cannot be detected with traditional clinical and radiographic methods [Bader et al., 2001; Ismail, 2004; Ko et al., 2008].

Caries prevention and fluoride

Frequent exposure to fluoride, optimal oral hygiene and a reduction in the intake of fermentable carbohydrates are important factors to be considered in caries prevention [Lingström et al., 2003; Selwitz et al., 2007]. The basic methods for preventing dental caries are generally the same, regardless of the tooth site and surface. However, some methods may be more suitable for certain areas. For example, the application of fissure sealants is a method recommended for caries prevention on occlusal surfaces [Mejàre et al., 2003], while fluoridated toothpicks, flosses and an interdental brush combined with fluoride gel are methods recommended for the approximal area [Kashani et al., 1998a; Särner et al., 2003; Särner et al., 2008].

The observed decline in dental caries in most industrialised countries over the last four decades can be attributed primarily to the daily use of fluoridated toothpaste [Bratthall et al., 1996; Marinho et al., 2003c; Twetman et al., 2003]. The bulk of modern research has confirmed the anticariogenic properties of fluoride and its key role in caries prevention [Featherstone, 1999; Marinho et al., 2003b]. The anticariogenic action of fluoride depends mainly on its ability to inhibit the demineralisation of enamel and dentine, to stimulate remineralisation [ten Cate, 1997; ten Cate et al., 1998; ten Cate, 1999; ten Cate et al., 2008] and to affect the metabolism of cariogenic bacteria [Selwitz et al., 2007; Wiegand et al., 2007; Stoodley et al., 2008]. Nowadays, brushing with fluoridated toothpaste twice a day as soon as the eruption of the first primary tooth takes place is highly recommended [Twetman et al., 2003; Alm, 2008]. In addition to toothpaste, a wide range of fluoridated products, such as mouthrinse solutions, gels, tablets, chewing gums, toothpicks and dental floss, is currently available.

Research has shown that the effect of fluoride-containing products, such as toothpaste and tablets, is less pronounced on approximal surfaces [Granath et al., 1978; Li et al., 1994; Øgaard et al., 1994]. The prevalence of approximal caries can be reduced by the frequent application of fluoride varnish [Moberg Sköld et al., 2005].

Miswaks and oral hygiene

Good oral hygiene habits can prevent or retard the development of caries and periodontal diseases [Axelsson et al., 2004]. Toothbrushes and toothpastes are the most widely used teeth cleaning tools. The toothbrush, which is relatively modern, was introduced in Europe around 300 years ago [Elvin-Lewis, 1980; Penick, 2004]. Historically, the first known oral hygiene device is the chewing stick. "Miswak" is an Arabic word meaning tooth cleaning stick and it has various local names in different Arabic dialects and countries. It is known as Miswak and Siwak in the Middle East, Mswaki in Tanzania, Mefaka in Ethiopia and Datun in India and Pakistan [Khoory, 1983; Hattab, 1997; Petersen and Mzee, 1998]. In English, it is known as the "toothbrush tree", "mustard plant", the "toothbrush tree of the Orient" and the "Persian toothbrush tree". The use of the chewing stick began more than 7,000 years ago. The Babylonians were the first to use it, followed by the Greeks and Romans and then the Jews, Egyptians and Muslims [Asadi and Asadi, 1997; Wu et al., 2001; Al-Otaibi, 2004]. The Japanese used Koyoji, while the Romans used Mastic to rub their teeth and the Jews used a kind of wooden stick called Qesam in Hebrew [Gerrit 1993].

Chewing sticks are used by 90% of Nigerian people and the inhabitants of rural regions of Tanzania and Zanzibar [Elvin-Lewis, 1980; Norton and Addy, 1989; Petersen and Mzee, 1998]. In Saudi Arabia, a large study of 1,155 patients, 65% were found to use chewing stick every day [Al-Otaibi et al., 2003b]. Another study by Guile et al., [1998] based on a sample of 3,117 people, reported chewing stick use by 50% of 15-year-old children. In India, more than 65% of the rural population and 43% of the urban population used chewing stick regularly [Boghani, 1978]. In Pakistan, more than 50% of the rural population used a chewing stick [Asadi and Asadi, 1997].

The Miswak material is harvested from a plant called Salvadora Persica or Are tree (synonymous with Araak). It is a small, upright, evergreen shrub with white branches and aromatic roots [Wu et al., 2001; Al-Otaibi, 2004], The roots, twigs and stems have been used for centuries for oral hygiene and are commonly used nowadays in the Middle East, as well as in Asia, Africa and South America [Elvin-Lewis, 1980; Eid and Selim, 1994; Wu et al., 2001].

Most chewing sticks are pencil-sized sticks, 15-20 cm long, with a diameter of 1-1.5 cm [Al-Sadhan et al., 1999; Wu et al., 2001; Al-Otaibi, 2004]. There are about 200 plant species that used for preparing brush sticks, of which more than 150 are found in Africa [Elvin-Lewis, 1982; Al-Otaibi, 2004] and the most widely used is *Salvadora Persica*, which is distributed geographically in Asia, Africa and the Middle East [Khoory, 1983; Wu et al., 2001]. They are prepared from the root, stem, twigs or bark of the trees. However, the plant is spongy and can easily be crushed between the teeth (Fig. 1A). Fig. 1B shows how one end of the stick is chewed or tapered until it becomes frayed into a brush. These sticks are sold in kiosks or small shops (Fig. 1C). In the Kingdom of Saudi Arabia, Miswaks are also available in most pharmacies in a ready-made hygienic air vacuum plastic pack (Fig. 3D). A Miswak and a toothbrush are similar in that they have bristles, which are used to remove plaque from tooth surfaces mechanically. Unlike a conventional toothbrush, the bristles of the Miswak lie in the same long axis as its handle. The angulation in the toothbrush enables it to adapt more easily to the buccal and occlusal surfaces, particularly in the posterior teeth [Danielsen et al., 1989].

The stick is usually chewed only briefly to fray the fibres and it is then used as a brush applied to the teeth, gums and tongue (Fig. 1B). It may be soaked in water or left in the mouth for a couple of minutes to stimulate salivation and enhance cleaning. It should be kept moist when not in use [Al-Sadhan et al., 1999; Almas and Al-Lafi, 1995]. With each use, worn bristles are snipped away and new bristles are prepared by further chewing or tapering [Mohammad and Turner, 1983; Wu et al., 2001].

For Muslims, it is customary to use the chewing stick prior to each prayer (five times a day). The Miswak should be freshly cut so that it is flexible, easily chewed and still rich in active constituents [Almas and Al-Lafi, 1995; Al-Otaibi, 2004]. The root should be whitish-brown in colour; a dark brown colour indicates that the Miswak is no longer fresh [Grant, 1990]. A very dry, hard Miswak can be expected to damage the gums and other oral tissues. If dry, the end should be soaked in fresh water for 24 hours. However, soaking for unduly long periods causes the loss of active constituents and diminishes the therapeutic properties but without any loss of the mechanical effects on the teeth [Almas and Al-Lafi, 1995; Al-Sadhan et al., 1999]. Before use, the end of the chewing stick should be washed with water. It is then chewed repeatedly until the fibres stand out like the bristles of a toothbrush. These fibres should be clipped off every 24 hours.

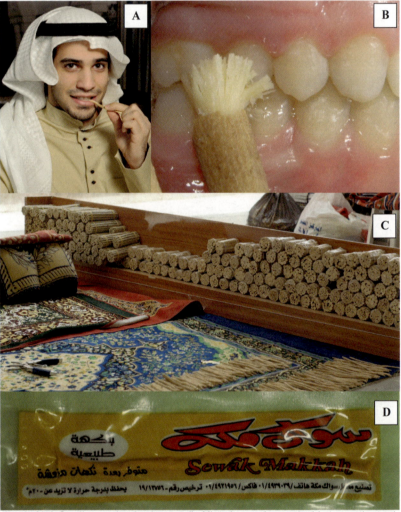

Fig. 1. A) A Saudi man showing how easily Miswaks can be crushed between the teeth. **B)** Miswaks become frayed like a brush when used orally. **C)** Kiosk or small shop sells Miswaks. **D)** A ready-made hygienic plastic vacuum-packed Miswak.

The value of chewing sticks is believed to lie in their mechanical cleansing action. Miswaks were also reported to inhibit the formation of dental plaque chemically and exert an antimicrobial effect on many oral bacteria [Al-Otaibi et al., 2003a; Al-Otaibi et al., 2004; Sofrata et al., 2007; Sofrata et al., 2008]. Several studies have reported that the prevalence and incidence of both dental caries and periodontal disease were low among chewing stick users compared with toothbrush and toothpaste users [Carl and Zambon, 1993; Schier and Cleaton-Jones, 1995; Sathananthan et al., 1996; Darout et al., 2000; Batwa et al., 2006]. A recent study in Saudi Arabia by Al-Otaibi et al., [2003a] found that the Miswak was more effective than toothbrushing in reducing plaque and gingivitis, when preceded by professional instructions on its correct application. Batwa et al., [2006] concluded that the Miswak was as effective as a toothbrush in reducing plaque on buccal teeth surfaces. Current studies frequently lack specific details relating to the time, duration and frequency of Miswak use, which prevents meaningful assessments of the mechanical cleansing role of Miswaks in oral health [Hardie and Ahmed, 1995a, b].

Extracts from the roots and stems of *Salvadora Persica* have shown antimicrobial activity, 5% sulphur as a major antimicrobial constituent [Ezmirly et al., 1979]. Al lafi and Ababneh, [1995] reported that trimethylamine, benzylisothiocyanate, B-sitosterol, m-anisic acid, salvadourea, chlorides, silica, large amounts of NaCl, KCl, sulphur, vitamin C, tannins, saponins, flavenoids and sterols, all of which are present in Miswaks, contributed to the Miswak's antibacterial effect on *Staphylococcus aureus* and other aerobic and anaerobic bacteria. Benzylisothiocyanate, a component exhibiting antiviral and antimycotic activity, has been shown to inhibit *in vitro* growth and acid production by mutans streptococci, but its mode of action has not been clearly delineated [Al-Bagieh et al., 1994]. The substantial amount of silica detected in *Salvadora Persica* ashes has been thought to contribute to the Miswak's mechanical action in plaque removal [Almas and Al-Lafi, 1995]. The potential contribution by fluoride was considered unlikely, as it is soluble and its total content in the Miswak, especially that released when soaked in water, is negligible (< 0.07 µg/ml) [Hattab, 1997; Wu et al., 2001; Al-Otaibi, 2004].

Despite increasing numbers of clinical surveys and epidemiological studies of chewing sticks and their oral health benefits, relatively few studies have looked into the antimicrobial effect of chewing stick extracts on oral pathogens associated with caries and periodontal disease. In 2004, Almas and Al-Zeid, [2004] conducted a clinical study to assess the antimicrobial activity of the Miswak and they revealed that mutans streptococci were more susceptible to Miswak antimicrobial activity than lactobacilli. Mouth rinsing with an aqueous extract of Miswaks significantly reduced the bacterial counts in salivary samples obtained up to 3 hours after rinsing [Gazi et al., 1992]. The extracts also inhibited glycolytic reactions by the salivary bacteria for up to 90 min post-rinsing. In a recent study by Almas et al., [2005], comparing the antimicrobial effect of a Miswak-based mouthwash with other commercially available non-alcohol mouth rinses, a mild reduction in mutans streptococci was noted.

The World Health Organisation (WHO) has recommended and encouraged the use of chewing sticks as an effective tool for oral hygiene [World Health Organisation, 1987]. With a better understanding of the properties, clinical effectiveness and the development of effective techniques with the emphasis on the frequency and thoroughness of the cleaning, chewing sticks may represent an equivalent or alternative instrument to the toothbrush for the prevention and control of dental diseases in developing countries [Al-Otaibi, 2004].

Fluoridation of toothpicks and other products

At the beginning of the 1980s, the idea of impregnating toothpicks in fluoride solutions stimulated two Norwegian researchers, [Mørch and Bjørvatn, 1981], who studied fluoride-impregnated toothpicks in the laboratory. The effect of fluoridated toothpicks was studied in a thesis by Kashani, [1998]. Toothpicks made of both birch and lime were found quickly to take up and release fluoride into the approximal area. Kashani and co-workers [Kashani et al., 1995; Kashani, 1998; Kashani et al., 1998b] carried out extensive studies on toothpicks impregnated in 1%, 2%, 3% and 4% NaF for 30 sec, 30 min or 3 days, which were used *in vivo* for 2 min. The results revealed that there was a clear dose-response effect and that the concentration of fluoride was highest during the first 5 min. Significantly higher values were found in saliva for toothpicks impregnated in 4% NaF compared with 1% and 2% NaF. *In vivo*, when impregnated toothpicks were compared with some other fluoride products like mouthrinse solution, tablets and dentifrice, the result found that the fluoride concentration in whole saliva increased up to 60 min.

A recent thesis at our department Särner, [2008] showed that there are large variations in the fluoride release from various fluoridated toothpicks and dental flosses. Treatment with a fluoridated toothpick or dental floss can be expected to produce elevated fluoride concentrations in the approximal area for up to 60 min. Another interesting method for administering fluoride into the approximal area is to use an interdental brush dipped in a fluoride gel [Särner et al., 2008].

Use of chewing sticks in the remineralisation of caries lesions

In individuals with a high caries risk, such as orthodontic patients, extra means of fluoride home care and professional fluoride application are recommended [Zimmer, 2001; SBU, 2002; Ellwood et al., 2008]. The demineralisation of enamel adjacent to the brackets is a clinical problem during treatment and even after debonding, as shown in Fig. 2. They develop as a result of dietary carbohydrate and acid production in plaque, resulting in an imbalance between the demineralisation and remineralisation of the enamel [Benson et al., 2004]. This is an interrupted process, with periods of remineralisation and demineralisation, depending on the state of the oral environment in terms of the prolonged accumulation and retention of bacterial plaque on the enamel surface, the standard of individual oral hygiene and the fluoride exposure [Featherstone, 2000; Aoba, 2004]. A white spot lesion (WSL) is the precursor of frank enamel caries. The white appearance of early enamel caries is due to an optical phenomenon, which is caused by mineral loss in the surface or subsurface enamel. Enamel crystal dissolution begins with subsurface demineralisation, creating pores between the enamel rods. The affected area is a consequence of both surface roughness and the loss of surface shine and alterations in internal reflection. This results in greater visual enamel opacity, since porous enamel scatters more light than sound enamel [Gorelick et al., 1982; Øgaard, 1989b]. The demineralisation process may encompass the full thickness of the enamel and some of the dentine before the relatively hyper-mineralised surface layer is actually lost.

It is generally accepted that the insertion of fixed orthodontic appliances creates stagnation areas for plaque and makes tooth cleaning more difficult. The irregular surfaces of brackets, bands, wires and other attachments also limit naturally occurring self-cleaning mechanisms, such as the movement of the oral musculature and saliva [Ng'ang'a and Øgaard, 1993]. This in turn encourages a lower plaque-pH in the presence of carbohydrates and accelerates the rate of plaque accumulation. These changes in the local environment appear to favour colonisation by aciduric bacteria, such as mutans streptococcus and lactobacilli. It has been reported that these levels can increase up to fivefold during orthodontic treatment [Sudjalim et al., 2006]. Since orthodontic treatment may result in temporary elevations in the number of cariogenic micro-organisms, the use of antimicrobials, such as chlorhexidine, may be justified in some patients [Derks et al., 2004].

It has been reported that there is a significant increase in the prevalence and severity of enamel demineralisation after orthodontic treatment when compared with untreated control subjects [Lovrov et al., 2007]. The overall prevalence of WSL among orthodontic patients has been reported to be anywhere between 50% and 96% [Gorelick et al., 1982; Øgaard et al., 1988; Gorton and Featherstone, 2003; Boersma et al., 2005]. Once active orthodontic treatment has been completed and the patient has been debonded, the demineralisation process is normally expected to decline due to positive changes in local environmental factors. Some WSL may remineralise and return to either normal or at least a visually acceptable appearance. On the other hand, some lesions may persist, leading to an aesthetically unacceptable result. In severe cases, restorative treatment may be required [Øgaard, 1989a; Sudjalim et al., 2006; Sudjalim et al., 2007].

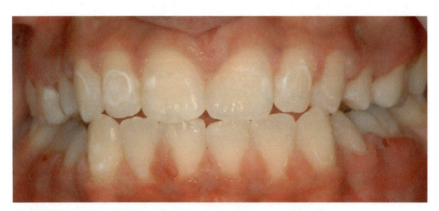

Fig. 2. White spot lesions after orthodontic treatment at debonding visit.

The overall management of WSL takes methods to prevent demineralisation and encourage remineralisation into consideration. Preventive measures play a pivotal role and are challenging, especially when treating patients with a high caries activity. In addition to regular professional oral hygiene visits, dietary control and the application of appropriate fluoride products, successful preventive strategies include oral health promotion, patient education and patient motivation.

From this point of view, the impregnation of chewing sticks with fluoride appears to be worth studying. This thesis was conducted to evaluate possible ways of fluoridating Miswaks, to study the fluoride release both *in vitro* and *in vivo* and to examine the effect of fluoridated Miswaks on remineralisation of white spot lesions (WSL).

Aims

General aim

The present thesis aimed at evaluating the uptake and release of the fluoride from fluoridated Miswaks *in vitro* and the oral fluoride retention and its effect *in vivo*.

Specific aims

1. To study the uptake and release of fluoride from fluoridated Miswaks both *in vitro* and *in vivo* (Papers I & II)
2. To evaluate the optimal and standard level of fluoride concentration in the fluoridated Miswak *in vivo* to be used on a daily basis (Paper II)
3. To evaluate the oral fluoride retention and concentration in whole saliva after using different concentrations of fluoridated Miswaks compared with brushing with fluoride toothpaste *in vivo* (Papers I, II & III)
4. To compare the oral fluoride retention and concentration after using fluoridated Miswaks in orthodontic patients before and after removal of their fixed appliances *in vivo* (Paper III)
5. To investigate the effect of fluoridated Miswaks on the remineralisation of white spot lesions (WSL), which have developed around orthodontic bands and brackets during orthodontic treatment *in vivo* (Paper IV)

Material and Methods

Study design

Paper I

The uptake and release of fluoride from fluoridated Miswaks in four different NaF concentrations and three different impregnation times were evaluated *in vitro* and *in vivo* in a clinical experimental study.

Paper II

The release of the fluoride from different NaF concentrations of fluoridated Miswaks was evaluated *in vitro* in two different test series (Series I & II) in an experimental study. The same products were tested to evaluate the oral fluoride retention *in vivo* compared with fluoride toothpaste as a control in a double-blind, randomised, cross-over experimental study.

Paper III

The effects of fluoride release and oral retention of six different home-care fluoride products were tested in orthodontic patients before and after the removal of their fixed appliances in a randomised, cross-over clinical study *in vivo*.

Paper IV

The remineralisation effect of fluoride released from fluoridated Miswaks on WSL in post-orthodontic patients was evaluated in a 6-week longitudinal, randomised, double-blind clinical study.

Subjects, test products and treatments

Paper I

In vitro. Three experimental series were conducted using 200 prepared Miswaks. In the first series, 120 pieces (10 pieces x 4 concentrations x 3 impregnation times) were impregnated in 1%, 2%, 3% and 4% NaF for 3 hours, 1 day and 3 days. A total of 12 different types of fluoridated Miswak were evaluated for both the uptake and release of fluoride. In the second series, 20 Miswaks were impregnated in 3% NaF for 1 day. The third series was identical to the second, except that the impregnation time was

21

prolonged to 3 days. The bark was separated from the pulp and the two parts placed in separate vials.

In vivo. Nine healthy adult volunteers, mean age 60 years, were recruited from the staff at the Institute of Odontology in Gothenburg. All the subjects were instructed not to use any fluoride-containing oral hygiene products and to reduce their intake of fluoride-containing food products to a minimum of 48 hours prior to each test occasion. They were not allowed to eat/drink, use tobacco or snuff or brush their teeth one hour before each test session. Three different fluoridated products were used: 1) Miswaks impregnated in 3% NaF for 1 day, 2) Miswaks impregnated in 3% NaF for 3 days and 3) 1 gram of fluoride toothpaste (containing 1450 ppm fluoride as NaF) applied to a toothbrush. The cover of the Miswak was first removed. It was then chewed for a short time and moved around the dentition to clean all the buccal and buccally oriented approximal surfaces for 2 min (Fig. 1A). Toothbrushing was carried in a normal manner for 2 min. For each individual, the tests were carried out at the same time of the day. There were a total of 27 visits for all patients, testing 3 products (two different fluoridated Miswaks and one regular fluoridated toothpaste) during an experimental period of 4 weeks.

Paper II

For both the *in vitro* and the *in vivo* experimental studies, a total of around 400 pieces of Miswak were used.

In vitro. Two series were performed using 200 prepared Miswaks. In the first, 100 pieces (50 old and 50 fresh) were impregnated in 0.01%, 0.1%, 0.5%, 1% and 3% NaF for one day and were used to evaluate the difference in fluoride release between old and fresh Miswaks. In the second series, a total of 100 pieces, selected randomly from 10 different stores (10/store), were impregnated in 0.5% NaF for one day and used to evaluate whether there were any differences in the fluoride release between the Miswaks that were purchased from 10 different stores.

In vivo. A total of 20 healthy adult volunteers were recruited from patients and the staff at the Institute of Odontology in Gothenburg. They participated in four series (called I-IV); in Series I and II, there were 10 healthy adults (6 men and 4 women) and, in Series III and IV, there were 10 other healthy adults (6 women and 4 men). All the subjects were instructed not to brush their teeth with fluoride-containing toothpaste on the day of the examination and not to eat or drink for at least 2 hours before the test. Five Miswaks, fluoridated in 0.01%, 0.1%, 0.5%, 1% and 3% NaF for 1 day (Series I), were tested to evaluate the "fluoride intake" when using a Miswak. The subject was instructed not to swallow any saliva but instead to spit into a beaker during this 2-min period and for the next 10 min. After this 2+10=12-min period, the patient finally rinsed his/her mouth with 20 ml of distilled water for 30 sec and spat it out into the same beaker. In the second (Series II), another five Miswaks impregnated in 0.01%, 0.1%, 0.5%, 1% and 3% NaF for 1 day were used to study the fluoride concentration in saliva after using a fluoridated Miswak for 2 min. Series III & IV were identical to Series I & II, except that a more narrow range of NaF impregnation solutions (0.05%, 0.1%, 0.2%, 0.3%, 0.4% and 0.5% NaF for 1 day) was used. Moreover, the subjects brushed with 1 g of fluoride toothpaste (containing 0.32% NaF) applied to a toothbrush.

Paper III

Nine healthy orthodontic patients (7 females and 2 males), with a mean age of 16 years (range 14-19), almost at the stage of debonding, were recruited from the specialist orthodontic clinics at the Institute of Odontology in Gothenburg. They used six different home-care fluoridated products before and after the removal of their fixed appliances. Each patient completed the 12 visits within 3 months. The products were: 1) toothpaste with 0.32% NaF (Pepsodent, Lever Fabergé, Stockholm, Sweden), 2) toothpaste with 1.1% NaF (Duraphat, Colgate-Palmolive, Glostrup, Denmark), 3) mouthrinse solution with 0.05% NaF (Dentan, Meda, Stockholm, Sweden), 4) mouthrinse solution with 0.2% NaF (Dentan, Meda), 5) Miswaks impregnated in 0.05% NaF for one day and 6) Miswaks impregnated for one day in 0.5% NaF. Prior to each test, the subjects chewed on paraffin wax for 5 min and rinsed with distilled water for 30 sec.

Toothpaste. 1 g of paste was applied to a wet toothbrush and the subject brushed his/her teeth for 2 min. After brushing, the remaining toothpaste was spat out and the mouth was rinsed with 5 ml of water for 5 sec.

Mouthrinse solution. 10 ml of the solution were swished around in the mouth for 2 min with active movements of the cheeks and lips.

Miswak. The cover was first removed and the participants then chewed on the stick for a short time (3-5 sec), before it was moved around the dentition to clean all the buccal tooth surfaces and all the buccally oriented approximal surfaces for 2 min.

Paper IV

Thirty-seven orthodontic patients (11 males and 26 females), with a mean age of 17.2 years, from three different dental hospitals in Jeddah, Saudi Arabia: 1) the King Fahad Armed Forces Hospital, 2) the King Faisal Specialist Hospital and Research Centre and 3) the King Fahad General Hospital were recruited after completion of their orthodontic treatment. The inclusion criterion was at least 2 WSL on both the left and right side of the dentition in the upper jaw, i.e. a minimum of 4 WSL/subject (total of 152 WSL in the test group and 140 WSL in the control group). Two different products were used: 1) fluoridated Miswaks impregnated in 0.5% NaF for one day and 2) non-fluoridated Miswaks (natural fresh Miswaks). The participants were randomly divided into two groups: 1) a test group with 19 patients using fluoridated Miswaks and 2) a control group with 18 patients using non-fluoridated Miswaks. The two types of Miswak were identical except for their fluoride content. An individual plastic mouth tray (Essix, Dentsply, Parkland, USA) covering half the dentition was used (Fig. 3). The tray was applied to the teeth immediately after toothbrushing and was kept in place, while using the Miswak and for a minimum of 30 min afterwards. The Miswaks were used 5 times/day. The WSL were scored using a DIAGNOdent pen, as well as the International Caries Detection and Assessment System (ICDAS II) index, at baseline and 2, 4 and 6 weeks after debonding.

The DIAGNOdent device has been studied extensively both *in vivo* and *in vitro* for detection of caries lesions on occlusal and smooth surfaces [Lussi et al., 1999; Shi et al., 2000; Attrill and Ashley, 2001; Lussi et al., 2001; Alwas-Danowska et al., 2002; Costa et al., 2002; Ouellet et al., 2002; Baseren and Gokalp, 2003; Cortes et al., 2003; Francescut and Lussi, 2003; Kordic et al., 2003; Bader and Shugars, 2004; Fung et al., 2004; Mendes et al., 2005]. Recent studies by Anttonen et al., [2003, 2004] and Sköld-Larsson et al., [2004] support the application of the method for detection and monitoring of caries. The DIAGNOdent has been tested *in vitro* for quantification of lesions adjacent to fixed orthodontic appliances [Staudt et al., 2004].

The International Caries Detection and Assessment System (ICDAS), based on visual inspection, was developed for use in clinical research, clinical practice and for epidemiological purposes [Pitts, 2004]. The system was intended to be feasible for use in epidemiological surveys and to detect cavitated and non-cavitated caries lesions with acceptable reliability [Pitts, 2004; Ismail et al., 2007].

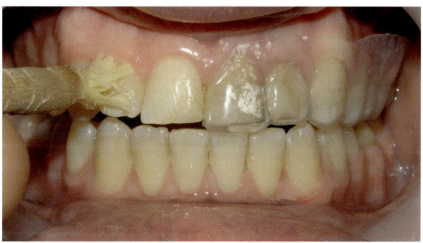

Fig. 3. Use of fluoridated Miswaks for cleaning the teeth with a custom-made mouth tray covering half the dentition in the upper jaw in Study IV. The cleaning was only performed in the non-covered area.

Miswaks preparation and fluoridating procedure

Fresh Miswaks bundles were purchased and transported from the Kingdom of Saudi Arabia to Sweden and kept in a refrigerator for 2 weeks prior to the start of each study. Each bundle contained 15-cm long sticks from the *Salvadora Persica* tree. From these bundles, five different sticks were selected randomly and cut with a scalpel into different lengths (3-4-cm long pieces). Fluoridation was carried out at Department of Cariology in Gothenburg for all four studies (I-IV). Fluoridated Miswaks were packed and transported back to Saudi Arabia one week prior to the start of Study IV.

Miswaks are natural products and there are great variations in size, diameter and colour (Fig. 4A). We tried to control for these factors, by visual inspection, in order to have all the specimens as similar as possible, especially with regard to size and weight (Fig. 4B). After cutting and coding, they were kept in distilled water for 6 hours (in order to clean them from dust). They were then dried in an oven at 40°C overnight

(Fig. 4C). For each concentration, Miswaks were placed in a vial with 500 ml of NaF solution for 3 hours, 1 day and 3 days in Paper I and for one day in Papers II-IV, i.e. with an excess of solution (Fig. 4D). After impregnation, the Miswaks were removed from the bottle (with forceps) and placed on paper at room temperature overnight in order to dry (Fig. 4E). They were packed in a clear plastic sealed nylon bag (Fig. 4F) and stored in a refrigerator to keep them clean.

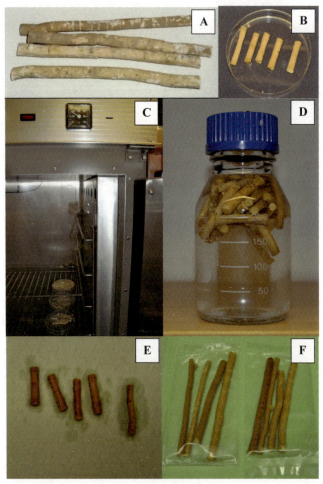

Fig. 4. A) Miswaks showing variations in size, colour and diameter. **B)** 3-cm-long pieces of Miswak cut to be as similar as possible. **C)** Drying of Miswaks in the oven at 40°C. **D)** Miswaks impregnated in NaF solution. **E)** Drying Miswaks after impregnation on paper at room temperature overnight. **F)** Packing Miswaks in a sealed clear plastic bag.

Scanning electron microscope (SEM)

One non-impregnated Miswak and one Miswak impregnated with 3% NaF were air-dried, spattered with gold and analysed in a Scanning Electron Microscope (SEM) (Leica S420; Leica Microsystems, Heidelberg, Germany, equipped with LEO Software 15XX) in order to examine the NaF crystal on the surface of the Miswak. Figures 5A and C show a magnified cross-section of the fluoridated Miswaks, showing clear multiple shiny dots representing NaF crystal deposition inside the pulp and on the bark of the Miswaks. Figures 5B and D show non-fluoridated Miswaks with no NaF crystals.

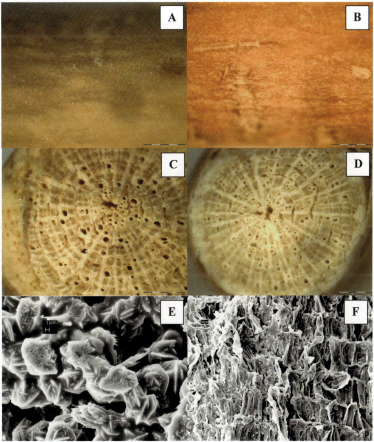

Fig. 5. A) White NaF crystal on the bark of a fluoridated Miswak. **B)** The bark of a non-fluoridated Miswak. **C)** Multiple shiny dots in a cross-section of a fluoridated Miswak showing a deposit of NaF crystals. **D)** Cross-section of a non-fluoridated Miswak. **E)** SEM of the outer surface (bark) of a fluoridated Miswak. **F)** SEM of the outer surface (bark) of a non-fluoridated Miswak.

SEM analysis images of a Miswak impregnated in 3% NaF is shown in Fig. 5E. There were "snowflake"-like crystals on the outer surface (bark) of the Miswak. However, the shape of these crystals looked different compared with NaF crystals found on a glass surface. Figure 5F shows SEM analysis images of a non-fluoridated Miswak. There were mesh-shaped fibres on the outer surface (bark) of the Miswak with no signs of any crystal deposits.

Sampling procedure

In vitro. After drying, each piece was transferred to a 20-ml bottle with 15 ml of distilled water and 1.5 ml of TISAB III solution (Orion Research, Boston, MA, USA). 0.3-ml aliquots were sucked up with a pipette on nine occasions (0, 1, 2, 5, 10, 15, 30, 40 and 60 min) and transferred to a 2-ml beaker covered with a lid. The samples were then kept in a refrigerator for up to one week before the fluoride analysis.

In vivo. Sampling of two approximal sites in Paper I (14/15 and 24/25) and in Paper III (15/16 and 24/25) was carried out before (0 min; baseline) and after 1, 3, 5, 7, 9, 15, 30 and 60 min after finishing the 2-min cleaning procedure. The sampling method according to Kashani et al. [1998] was used. Small triangle-shaped paper points (base: 1.5 mm; length: 5 mm) were inserted in the approximal area for 30 sec in order to suck up around 4 µl of saliva (Fig. 6). The paper points were then transferred to Eppendorf tubes, containing 200 µl of de-ionised water and 20 µl of TISAB III buffer solution (dilution 10:1; Thermo Electron, Waltham, Mass., USA).

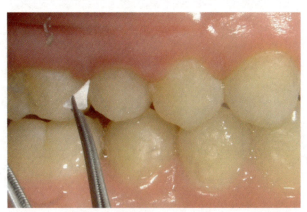

Fig. 6. Sampling of approximal fluid with triangular paper points.

In Papers II & III, resting whole saliva was collected just before (0-min sample; baseline) and after 1, 3, 5, 10, 15, 30 and 60 min, making 8 samples/test. For Paper II, a total of 800 saliva samples were collected for the *in vivo* study (9 subjects x 5 products x 1 site x 8 time points x 2 series). For Paper III, a total of 864 saliva samples were collected (9 subjects x 6 products x 1 site x 8 time points x 2 occasions).

Fluoride analysis

All the samples were analysed blind in terms of the subjects and methods. The same technician analysed all the samples.

In vitro. The fluoride concentration was determined by means of a fluoride-sensitive electrode connected to an expandable ion analyser (Orion Research, Boston, MA, USA). Ionic strength was stabilised by adding a buffer solution (TISAB III) according to the manufacturer's instructions. All the analyses were performed using standard solutions from 0.526 μM (0.01 ppm) to 5.26 mM (100 ppm) fluoride. The detection level of fluoride was approximately 0.5 μM.

In vivo study. Each paper point was transferred to a 0.5-ml Eppendorf tube, containing 200 μl of distilled water and 20 μl of TISAB III (Orion Research). The absorbed fluoride was allowed to diffuse from the paper point into the solution for 24 hours in a refrigerator. Prior to analysis, the samples were thoroughly mixed by vibration for 10 sec. The fluoride concentration was then analysed using the ion-specific electrode.

Ethical considerations

The first three studies (I-III) were approved by the Ethics Committee at the University of Gothenburg. Study IV was approved by the Ethics Committee at 1) the King Fahad Armed Forces Hospital, 2) the King Faisal Specialist Hospital and Research Centre and 3) the King Fahad General Hospital. Both verbal and written information about the individual studies was given to the subjects. Written informed consent was obtained from all the subjects prior to the start of each study. All the subjects were coded when entering the individual studies and the statistical analyses were performed with unidentifiable data.

Statistical methods

The sample size was based on a simple power analysis that was performed before the start of each study (Papers I-III) and from earlier studies by Kashani et al., [1998] and Särner et al., [2003]. Even if statistically significant differences were obtained with six individuals, it was nonetheless decided to include 9-10 subjects in all the *in vivo* series.

In Papers I & II, the area under the curve (AUC) was calculated using the KaleidaGraph software program version 4.0 (Synergy Software, Reading, Pa., USA) for each individual and each treatment. Statistical comparisons were made using two-way analysis of variance (ANOVA), $p < 0.05$ was considered statistically significant. In Paper II, an unpaired t-test was applied to the 60-min fluoride values *in vitro* in order to compare old and fresh Miswaks, as well as Miswaks from different stores.

In Paper III, means and standard deviations were calculated for each F product with and without the fixed orthodontic appliances. AUC was measured then the mean differences between the AUC values with and without orthodontic appliances and between the various products were compared using a paired t-test ($p < 0.05$ was considered to be statistically significant). Statistical comparisons using three-way analysis of variance (ANOVA) were also performed, which confirmed the result of the paired t-test.

In Paper IV, a power analysis was performed before the start of the study and a sample size of 17 patients/group was suggested. Means and standard deviations were calculated for each visit and patient for both ICDAS II and DIAGNOdent pen measurements. The mean values were calculated for the teeth in one and the same quadrant. The mean changes (Δ) for baseline vs. 6 weeks for the covered and a non-covered side were analysed using a paired t-test. For comparisons between the test and control group, a non-paired t-test was used. As a multiple t-test was used, the correlation between the ICDAS II index score and the DIAGNOdent readings at baseline and at 6 weeks was analysed using Pearson's correlation coefficient.

Results

Studies I & II

In vitro. A clear dose-response effect with respect to fluoride concentration and impregnation time was found; the higher the NaF solution used and the longer the impregnation time, the greater the release of fluoride (Paper I). Moreover, fresh Miswaks produced a slightly higher fluoride release than old Miswaks, especially at high NaF impregnation concentrations (i.e. at 1% and 3% NaF). However, there were no statistically significant differences between fresh and old Miswaks at 60 min for any of the five NaF concentrations (Paper II).

The release of fluoride was linear with time, but a more rapid release during the first 10 min, especially when impregnated in 3% and 4% NaF, was found in Studies I & II (Fig. 7).

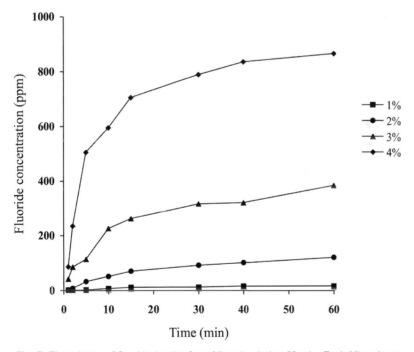

Fig. 7. The release of fluoride *in vitro* from Miswaks during 60 min. Each Miswak was impregnated in 1%, 2%, 3% or 4% NaF for 3 days and dried and placed in 5 ml of distilled water (mean values of 10 samples/test).

The bark released more fluoride than the pulp, but both parts produced a fast, high release, especially during the first 10 min. The results for impregnation in 3% NaF for 3 days showed parallel curves for the bark and the pulp, as shown in Fig. 8.

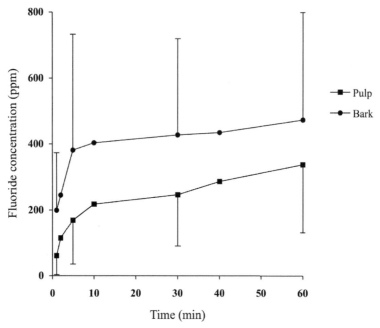

Fig. 8. The release of fluoride from the bark and the pulp of Miswaks impregnated in 3% NaF for 3 days (mean values of 20 samples/test). The standard deviation in one direction is given for every second value.

The differences in the weight of dried Miswaks before and after 3 hours' impregnation with NaF solution are shown in Table 1. The higher the NaF concentration used, the greater the uptake of fluoride by the Miswaks (Papers I & II).

Table 1. The weight (in grams) of 3-cm Miswaks after drying before and after impregnation in NaF solution for 3 hours and the difference, which indicates the uptake of NaF (mean values ± SD of 10 pieces/test).

NaF concentration	Difference (uptake) Between before and after impregnation
1%	0.20±0.04
2%	0.24±0.03
3%	0.42±0.11
4%	0.47±0.06

In vivo. For Study I, the fluoride concentration in the approximal area was elevated during the entire 30-min period and the AUC was twice as high for the Miswaks impregnated for 3 days compared with 1 day and four times higher compared with fluoride toothpaste ($p < 0.05$ and $p < 0.01$ respectively). The mean salivary fluoride concentration and the AUC values of Miswaks impregnated in 0.1-0.3% NaF produced about the same fluoride level as brushing with fluoride toothpaste (Fig. 9). The mean AUC in Series II was twice as high for the Miswaks impregnated in 3% NaF compared with 0.5% NaF ($p < 0.0001$) and four times higher compared with 0.1% NaF ($p < 0.0001$). In Series IV, the mean AUC was three times as high for Miswaks impregnated in 0.5% NaF compared with 0.05% NaF and twice as high compared with 0.1% NaF.

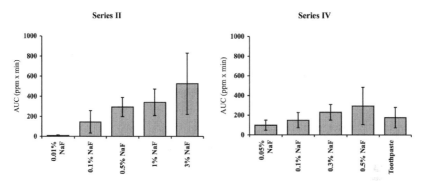

Fig. 9. The AUC values (mean and SD; n=10) in saliva *in vivo* from Series II (0.01%, 0.1%, 0.5%, 1% and 3% NaF) and Series IV (0.05%, 0.1%, 0.3%, 0.5% and toothpaste; the data from 0.2% and 0.4% are not shown).

The mean ± SD for the oral "fluoride intake", which is expressed as mg of fluoride for 6 of the 11 different NaF impregnation solutions, are shown in Table 2. Approximately 27-29 ml of saliva were collected during the 12 min, including the final mouthrinse with 20 ml of water. The calculated "fluoride intake" increased at higher NaF impregnation concentrations. At 0.1% NaF, it was a mean of 0.21 mg of fluoride (range 0.06-0.44) and, at 0.5% NaF, about twice as much, i.e. 0.39 mg of fluoride (range 0.21-0.61).

Table 2. The results from Series I and III *in vivo*. Both the total volume of saliva (ml), collected during 10+2=12 min, and the fluoride concentration (ppm) in saliva, including a mouth rinse with 20 ml of water, are shown. The "fluoride intake" was calculated as ml saliva x ppm fluoride and expressed as mg fluoride (mean ± SD and range of 10 individuals).

Impregnation solution (NaF)	Saliva + water rinse		"Fluoride intake" (mg F)[*]	
	Volume (ml)	F (ppm)	Mean ± SD	Range
0.1%	27.7±4.8	7.7±3.6	0.21±0.11	0.06-0.44
0.5%	28.1±5.7	14.0±5.6	0.39±0.13	0.21-0.61
3%	29.1±5.0	31.1±17.1	0.91±0.50	0.22-1.80

[*]Calculated as volume (ml) x ppm F / 1000 = mg F

Study III

Figure 10 shows the means and standard deviations of AUC in approximal saliva from the patients with orthodontic appliances; the six fluoride products are given in ranking order. 0.5% NaF-impregnated Miswaks produced the highest fluoride values, which was significantly higher compared with the other products ($p < 0.05$).

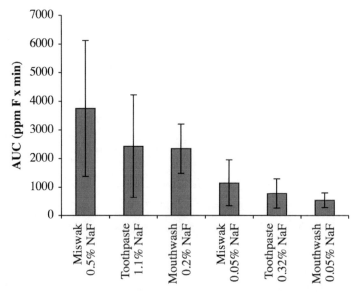

Fig. 10. The AUC values (mean ± SD) of the fluoride concentration in approximal fluid (mesial 25) from six different fluoride products, arranged in order from the highest to the lowest, in patients (n=9) wearing fixed orthodontic appliances.

Generally, in all the tests, the numerically highest fluoride release was mesial 25, followed by mesial 16. Using 0.5% NaF-impregnated Miswaks, both with and without orthodontic appliances, resulted in the highest fluoride retention in approximal saliva, especially at mesial 25, with statistically significant differences compared with all the other F products ($p < 0.001$).

The mean the AUC values with orthodontic appliances for 0.2% NaF mouthrinse solution, 1.1% NaF toothpaste and 0.5% NaF Miswaks are shown in Fig. 11. The fluoride concentration was high, especially during the first 10 min; there were no significant differences between the three sampling sites, except for Miswaks, which obtained higher values at the two approximal sites than in whole saliva ($p < 0.05$). Both the fluoride concentration and the AUC were about one and a half times higher for 0.5% NaF-impregnated Miswaks compared with 0.2% NaF mouthrinse solution and 0.5% NaF toothpaste ($p < 0.05$).

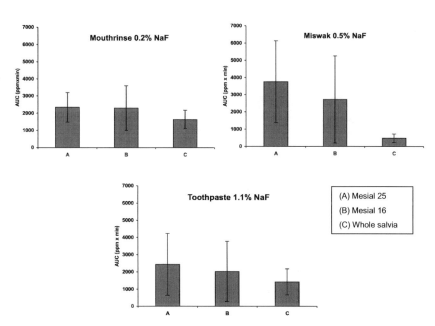

Fig. 11. Mean values (n=9) of the AUC values (0–60 minutes) both in saliva and at two approximal sites after using three fluoride products (0.2% NaF mouthrinse, 1.1% NaF toothpaste and 0.5% NaF-impregnated Miswaks) in orthodontic patients with fixed appliances.

Study IV

Figures 12 show the means and standard deviations of the readings from the DIAGNOdent pen at baseline and after 6 weeks for the non-covered quadrants. There was a gradual decrease for non-covered surfaces treated with fluoridated Miswaks in the test group (p < 0.0001). In the control group, the values stayed more or less the same. The result was the same with the International Caries Detection and Assessment System (ICDAS II) index values. It was found that the DIAGNOdent values correlated well with the ICDAS II clinical index (r=0.76). Thus, the progression/regression of WSL can be registered by both methods, even during such a short period as 6 weeks.

DIAGNOdent pen reading

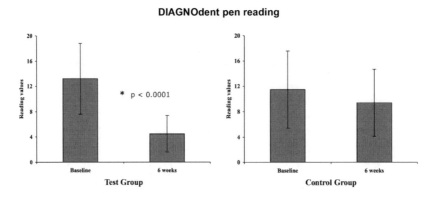

Fig. 12. Means and standard deviations of the DIAGNOdent pen readings for non-covered quadrants in the test (n=19) and control (n=18) groups at baseline and at 6 weeks.

Fig. 13A & B show an example of intra-oral clinical photographs taken for one patient in the control and one in the test groups both at baseline and at 6 weeks, illustrating the remineralising effect after using fluoridated Miswaks on WSL (test group) compared to non-fluoridated Miswaks (control group).

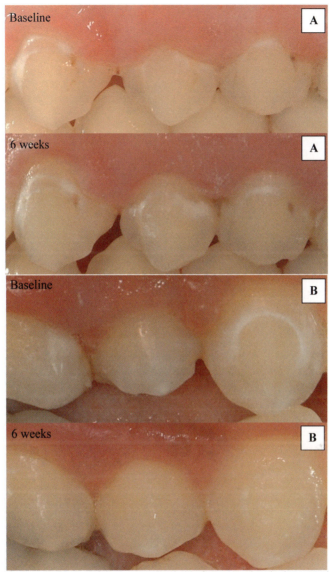

Fig. 13. A) Photos of the non-covered side for one patient in the control group showing no improvement of the WSL from baseline to 6 weeks after using non-fluoridated Miswaks. **B)** Photos of the non-covered side for one patient in the test group showing the WSL improvement from baseline to 6 weeks after using fluoridated Miswaks.

Discussion

This thesis was based on the concept that chewing sticks are frequently utilised in many countries around the world for cleaning purposes and are often used up to 5 times/day in Arabic countries. The prevalence of dental caries is high in different countries like Saudi Arabia [Alamoudi et al., 1996; Al-Shammery, 1999; Gandeh and Milaat, 2000; Wyne et al., 2001; Amin and Al-Abad, 2008]. In order to reduce and prevent dental caries in these countries, it may be interesting to study the idea of fluoridating Miswaks in order to have a dual effect, combining the mechanical cleaning effect and the anticariogenic effect achieved through fluoride release into the oral cavity.

In the present series of studies, the effect of fluoridated Miswaks was investigated in terms of the uptake and release of fluoride (Papers I & II), the fluoride clearance in the saliva and oral fluoride retention (Paper II), oral fluoride retention with and without orthodontic appliances (Paper III) and the remineralisation effect on white spot lesions "WSL" (Paper IV). Data from Papers I-IV revealed that Miswaks were generally suitable for both the uptake and release of NaF. This is in agreement with previous studies of fluoridated toothpicks [Mørch and Bjørvatn, 1981; Petersson et al., 1994; Kashani et al., 1995; Särner et al., 2003; Särner et al., 2008]. The fluoride uptake of Miswaks impregnated in 3% NaF for 3 hours in the present study was twice as high as the Miswaks impregnated in 1% NaF. As fluoride is released rapidly, this indicates that the fairly simple diffusion of NaF occurs through the surface (bark) into the Miswak pulp. This finding was confirmed in Study I, when fluoride release from the bark and the pulp was analysed separately.

The variation in the uptake and release of fluoride depends on several factors, such as the size, nature and degree of porosity within the Miswak. Mørch and Bjørvatn, [1981] suggested that a chemical reaction between fluoride and various organic or inorganic substances present in wood might take place and protect or inhibit the release of fluoride. In comparison to other products, it is not possible for technical reasons to assess the maximum fluoride content incorporated in a specific product. Fluoride incorporation probably occurs in both the bark and pulp of the Miswak. It appears that NaF crystals are absorbed to some extent within the Miswaks and fluoride is released intra-orally from the pulp after using the Miswak for 2 min and diminishes after 1 hour (Papers I-III). The release of fluoride from the bark of the Miswak was found to be higher than that from the pulp (bristles), but both parts produced a high, rapid fluoride release, especially during the first 10 min. The reason for this could be that the bark is thin and more porous, which may be due to the fact that a Miswak is originally the root of a plant, which is characterised by water absorption (Fig. 3).

There was a clear dose-response effect with respect to both the fluoride concentration and the impregnation time (Papers I&II). The higher the NaF concentration, the more fluoride that was absorbed, leading to more fluoride release from the Miswak, as found in studies of fluoridated toothpicks [Petersson et al., 1994; Kashani et al., 1995; Kashani, 1998; Särner et al., 2003; Särner et al., 2008]. High concentrations, such as 3% or 4% NaF solutions, were used for the impregnation of Miswaks in Papers I & II and produced a fluoride release that was 4-5 times higher compared with the toothpaste (0.32% NaF) when calculated as AUC. On the other hand, lower concentrations, such as 0.05% and 0.5% NaF solutions, were used in Papers II & III and produced a lower fluoride release. Miswaks impregnated in 4% NaF solution for 3 days displayed a very high level of fluoride release compared with any other fluoridated product, in addition to demonstrating a whitish layer consisting of NaF crystals (unpublished observations). To avoid this whitish discoloration of Miswaks, it is suggested to use Miswaks impregnated in 0.1% or 0.5% NaF for one day (Paper II).

The total uptake of fluoride in Miswaks impregnated in 4% NaF solution for 3 hours is about 0.47 mg (Paper I). About 60-70% of this fluoride was released after 1 hour of storage in water. The in vivo release is, however, much lower because the Miswak is used in the mouth for a much shorter time than one hour. In spite of the large uptake, a fair amount of fluoride is still released and swallowed during the use of Miswaks in the mouth. For this reason, only the bristle part of the Miswak should be in contact with the tooth surface and only part of the bark.

In Study II, fresh Miswaks released slightly more fluoride than old ones, even if the difference was not statistically significant. Both types are sold on the open market, but the fresh Miswaks are softer, taste better, are more flexible and somewhat more expensive. Moreover, there was a large difference in fluoride release from Miswaks purchased from different stores, with a factor of around 2. The reason for this variation could be that some of the stores sell fresh Miswaks, while others sell older types. The difference may also depend on the properties of the Miswak itself, even if we tried to control for both the size and weight of the pieces.

Large surface areas of the bristles of the Miswaks are in contact with the tooth surface during brushing, which means that a great deal of the released fluoride can then be subsequently swallowed. In Study II, Miswaks impregnated for one day in 0.5% NaF produced a mean "fluoride retention" of 0.39 mg of fluoride. If the Miswak is to be used five times a day, around 2 mg of fluoride will be swallowed every day. The daily fluoride intake of an adult has been estimated to be around 1-2 mg from food and fluoride toothpaste [Villa et al.]. This amount is considered safe for an adult from a toxicological point of view. However, for safety reasons and due to individual variations, the recommended impregnation is with 0.1% NaF, with a net intake of 0.21x5≈1 mg fluoride/day.

Previous studies of various fluoride products have usually involved measurements of the fluoride content of the whole saliva and plaque, but very few data on fluoride in the approximal area are available. Generally, the fluoride concentration values for all fluoridated products and for all patients with fixed orthodontic appliances showed higher fluoride retention values with than without the appliances. In Papers I & III, the fluoride concentration at various approximal sites measured after using fluoridated Miswaks, dentifrices and mouthrinse solutions. Fluoridated Miswaks was equivalent or superior to the other products. The result was that 0.5% fluoridated Miswaks were the best at delivering fluoride directly into the approximal area. In Paper III, 0.5% NaF Miswaks retained 1.5 times more fluoride than the 0.2% NaF rinsing solution and 0.5% NaF toothpaste in the approximal saliva. The advantage of Miswaks is that there is no need for post-brushing water rinsing, as there is after using toothpaste, and this could explain why fluoride retention in the approximal area is higher than with other fluoridated products. Several studies have reported the caries preventive effect of rinsing with fluoride mouthwash [Fure et al., 1998; Marinho et al., 2003a; Marinho et al., 2004b,a; Twetman et al., 2004]. A higher salivary fluoride concentration interproximally when using fluoride mouthrinses is attributed to better accessibility and spread, especially between brackets and wires, when compared with other fluoridated products. This is in agreement with the study by Särner et al., [2003], which showed that rinsing with 0.2% NaF resulted in higher approximal fluoride concentrations compared with fluoridated toothpicks and dental flosses.

The combined mechanical cleaning effect (achieved by the Miswak bristles) and the chemical effect of the fluoride impregnation regimens in the treatment and prevention of WSL were investigated in Paper IV. When it came to the remineralisation effect on WSL, fluoridated Miswaks were superior to non-fluoridated Miswaks. This difference may be due to fluoride release from the fluoridated Miswaks (chemical effect), the mechanical cleaning effect or both. The DIAGNOdent and clinical index methods were included in the study in order to compare them with one another. The study indicated that the DIAGNOdent provided a consistent performance and reliability as found previously by several studies [Lussi et al., 1999; Shi et al., 2000; Costa et al., 2002; Baseren and Gokalp, 2003; Cortes et al., 2003]. It could therefore be suitable for the longitudinal monitoring of caries lesions and subsequently aid in clinical decision-making with respect to the management of orthodontically induced smooth surface lesions. All the WSL in Study IV were also examined visually during the de-bonding visit and 6 weeks later. The differences between the clinical index readings at baseline and at the final examination were statistically significant. The clinical index correlated well with the DIAGNOdent values (r=0.76). The DIAGNOdent pen thus offered a possible means of detecting and quantifying minor changes that had occurred during the 6-week study period. These findings confirm the results of previous studies applying the DIAGNOdent method [Al-Khateeb et al., 1998; Aljehani et al., 2004; Bamzahim et al., 2004]. The advantage of the pen is that it is easy to carry, accurate, reproducible and the readings can be shown to the patient and may thus have a pedagogic value. On the other hand, it is expensive and time consuming. The advantages of using the ICDAS II are that it is easy to use, inexpensive and less time consuming. However, it is more subjective and less informative for the patient.

WSL that form around brackets during orthodontic treatment may possibly be remineralised over a relatively short period of time, as shown in Study IV. Other studies have reported longer periods of time that may extend to some years [Øgaard et al., 1988]. In our study, the test group patients were provided with fluoride toothpaste for use twice daily, combined with fluoridated Miswaks 5 times/day. The remineralisation is thus a combination of the cleaning effect of the Miswaks and their fluoride release. Since the control group was also given fluoride toothpaste and was using non-fluoridated Miswaks, the remineralisation of WSL can be mainly attributed to the fluoride release from the Miswaks. The slight regression of WSL in the covered sites in the subjects using the fluoridated Miswaks indicated that the mouth tray did not totally prevent fluoride from reaching the buccal surfaces. However, the effect was still stronger on the treated sites.

Several studies have assessed the presence of WSL by using photographic techniques. However, there are difficulties in achieving consistency in lightning, reflection and angulation. In Study IV, the light was standardised by using a ring flash with cross-polarisation filters and by fixing the focal length distance of the lens at 50 cm. In spite of this, it was not possible to obtain identical photos in order to score the WSL in an optimal way.

The successful fluoride impregnation of Miswaks can be efficiently incorporated in future community-targeted preventive programmes, especially in countries where Miswak use is common or a tradition. The advantages of fluoridated Miswaks as an alternative to the toothbrush are that it is inexpensive, readily available in both urban and rural areas, easy to carry, has medicinal properties, is hygienic and its use is not limited to the bathroom. On the other hand, accessibility to the lingual surfaces of the posterior teeth may be problematic when using a Miswak, as its bristles lie in the same long axis as its handle, as different from the toothbrush. In addition, specific written instructions should be given to the patient to avoid potential damage to the gingival tissues (gingival recession).

More extensive research on fluoridated Miswaks as a preventive regimen, should be applied in large populations such as schoolchildren, especially in countries where its use is very common, such as Saudi Arabia. In addition, it should be compared with fluoride toothpaste and mouthrinse. Taking account of the availability of plastic-packed chewing sticks in various pharmacies around Saudi Arabia, a clever way to commercialise the fluoridated Miswak in a more modern and hygienic fashion would be to introduce it in the market with special protective carriers, thereby facilitating its transport and keeping it fresh and clean.

Conclusions

The main conclusion from this series of studies is that fluoridated Miswaks are suitable vehicles for the uptake and release of fluoride both *in vitro* and *in vivo*. More specifically, the conclusions are as follows:

- The uptake and release of fluoride from fluoridated Miswaks both *in vitro* and *in vivo* are rapid processes (Papers I-II and III).
- Miswaks impregnated in 0.1% to 0.5% NaF for one day could be considered the "optimum level" with respect to both the fluoride concentration in saliva and the "fluoride retention" (Papers II-IV).
- The oral "fluoride retention" increased at higher NaF impregnation concentrations. At 0.1% NaF, it was a mean of 0.21 mg F and, at 0.5% NaF, it was 0.39 mg fluoride. Miswaks impregnated in 0.1% to 0.3% NaF produced about the same salivary fluoride level in saliva as brushing with fluoride toothpaste containing 0.32% NaF (Paper II).
- The oral fluoride retention was higher for all fluoride products when the patients were wearing fixed orthodontic appliances (Paper III).
- Fluoridated Miswaks impregnated with 0.5% NaF have a remineralisation effect on WSL compared with non-fluoridated Miswaks (Paper IV).

Acknowledgements

All praise to *Allah* Almighty (My Lord). First and foremost, I would like to thank *Allah* Almighty, the Generous, for making my dream come true.

I would like to express my sincere gratitude to everyone who has supported me during this strenuous journey.

First of all, Professor *Dowen Birkhed*, Head of the Department of Cariology at Sahlgrenska Academy, University of Gothenburg, my main supervisor, co-author, Swedish father and friend. I am very grateful to you for giving me the opportunity to be your PhD student. This privilege has undoubtedly nourished my research spirit. From day one, your guidance, patience, endless encouragement and fatherly care have provided me with a paramount source of will and power to work very hard to achieve only the best. Thank you for your optimistic attitude to life, which has opened doors of solutions to issues that might have seemed impossible to solve. I will be grateful to you forever. Without you, *Dowen*, this thesis would never have been achieved.

Professor *Peter Lingström*, my supervisor and co-author, for your constant kind support and insightful guidance. You were always available, shared your expertise and gave constructive criticism, which was extremely valuable in realising this thesis.

Associate Professor *Heidrun Kjellberg*, my supervisor and co-author. Thank you for your visionary approach and vast expertise and knowledge, which have inspired and guided me throughout my clinical training years. The orthodontist I have proudly become is, I hope, the rewarding harvest of your dedication to my education.

In addition I would like to thank the following people:

Emerita Professor *Birgit Thilander*, for her exceptional and valuable criticism, advice and availability, despite her tremendous responsibilities and duties.

Dr. Meshari Al-Otaibi, Kingdom of Saudi Arabia, for introducing me to the field of research on Miswaks.

Dr. Tommy Johnsson, for his statistical assistance.

Mrs Ann-Britt Lundberg and *Mrs. Ann-Charlott Börjesson,* for their excellent technical assistance at the Department of Cariology.

Orthodontic assistant *Monica Melin*, for her superb handling and organisation of patients' appointments and clinical assistance.

Elena Linder, at the Department of Periodontology, for assisting with the scanning electron microscopy.

Christina Eklund, at the Department of Oral microbiology, for assisting with imaging of scanning microscopy.

Jeanette Kliger, for her excellent revision of the English text.

My colleagues and friends at the Departments of Cariology and Orthodontics, for their support and friendship.

The Ministry of Higher Education in Saudi Arabia, along with Dammam University, Kingdom of Saudi Arabia, for fully funding my thesis.

I am forever indebted to my family: *Soha,* my wonderful wife, *Jude,* my lovely princess, for providing a loving atmosphere, extreme support, understanding, endless patience and encouragement throughout my research journey

Lastly, and most importantly, I wish to thank my dearly beloved parents, *Ali* and *Siham*. Also my brothers and sisters, *Mohamed Saleh*, *Yasser*, *Nawal* and *Ohoud*. I am who I am because of what they have done in raising me, supporting me and emphasising and respecting the nobility and privilege of being a researcher. To them, I dedicate this thesis. To my beloved father- and mother-in-law, *Mohamed Obaid* and *Shadia*. For their constant support and love at all times.

References

Al lafi T, Ababneh H: The effect of the extract of the miswak (chewing sticks) used in Jordan and the Middle East on oral bacteria. Int Dent J 1995;45:218-222.

Al Sadhan RI, Almas K. Miswak (chewing stick): a cultural and scientific heritage. Saudi Dent J 1999;11: 80-87.

Al-Bagieh NH, Idowu A, Salako NO: Effect of aqueous extract of miswak on the in vitro growth of Candida albicans. Microbios 1994;80:107-113.

Al-Khateeb S, Forsberg CM, de Josselin de Jong E, Angmar-Månsson B: A longitudinal laser fluorescence study of white spot lesions in orthodontic patients. Am J Orthod Dentofacial Orthop 1998;113:595-602.

Al-Otaibi M: The miswak (chewing stick) and oral health. Studies on oral hygiene practices of urban Saudi Arabians. Swed Dent J Suppl 2004:2-75.

Al-Otaibi M, Al-Harthy M, Gustafsson A, Johansson A, Claesson R, Angmar-Månsson B: Subgingival plaque microbiota in Saudi Arabians after use of miswak chewing stick and toothbrush. J Clin Periodontol 2004;31:1048-1053.

Al-Otaibi M, Al-Harthy M, Söder B, Gustafsson A, Angmar-Månsson B: Comparative effect of chewing sticks and toothbrushing on plaque removal and gingival health. Oral Health Prev Dent 2003a;1:301-307.

Al-Otaibi M, Zimmerman M, Angmar-Månsson B: Prevailing oral hygiene practices among urban Saudi Arabians in relation to age, gender and socio-economic background. Acta Odontol Scand 2003b;61:212-216.

Al-Shammery AR: Caries experience of urban and rural children in Saudi Arabia. J Public Health Dent 1999;59:60-64.

Alamoudi N, Salako NO, Massoud I: Caries experience of children aged 6-9 years in Jeddah, Saudi Arabia. Int J Paediatr Dent 1996;6:101-105.

Aljehani A, Tranaeus S, Forsberg CM, Angmar-Månsson B, Shi XQ: In vitro quantification of white spot enamel lesions adjacent to fixed orthodontic appliances using quantitative light-induced fluorescence and DIAGNOdent. Acta Odontol Scand 2004;62:313-318.

Alm A: On dental caries and caries-related factors in children and teenagers. Swed Dent J Suppl 2008:7-63.

Almas K, Al-Lafi TR: The natural toothbrush. World Health Forum 1995;16:206-210.

Almas K, Al-Zeid Z: The immediate antimicrobial effect of a toothbrush and miswak on cariogenic bacteria: A clinical study. J Contemp Dent Pract 2004;5:105-114.

Almas K, Skaug N, Ahmad I: An in vitro antimicrobial comparison of miswak extract with commercially available non-alcohol mouthrinses. Int J Dent Hyg 2005;3:18-24.

Alwas-Danowska HM, Plasschaert AJ, Suliborski S, Verdonschot EH: Reliability and validity issues of laser fluorescence measurements in occlusal caries diagnosis. J Dent 2002;30:129-134.

Amin TT, Al-Abad BM: Oral hygiene practices, dental knowledge, dietary habits and their relation to caries among male primary school children in Al Hassa, Saudi Arabia. Int J Dent Hyg 2008;6:361-370.

Anttonen V, Seppä L, Hausen H: Clinical study of the use of the laser fluorescence device DIAGNOdent for detection of occlusal caries in children. Caries Res 2003;37:17-23.

Anttonen V, Seppä L, Hausen H: A follow-up study of the use of DIAGNOdent for monitoring fissure caries in children. Community Dent Oral Epidemiol 2004;32:312-318.

Aoba T: Solubility properties of human tooth mineral and pathogenesis of dental caries. Oral Dis 2004;10:249-257.

Asadi SG, Asadi ZG: Chewing sticks and the oral hygiene habits of the adult Pakistani population. Int Dent J 1997;47:275-278.

Attrill DC, Ashley PF: Occlusal caries detection in primary teeth: A comparison of DIAGNOdent with conventional methods. Br Dent J 2001;190:440-443.

Axelsson P, Nyström B, Lindhe J: The long-term effect of a plaque control program on tooth mortality, caries and periodontal disease in adults. Results after 30 years of maintenance. J Clin Periodontol 2004;31:749-757.

Bader JD, Shugars DA: A systematic review of the performance of a laser fluorescence device for detecting caries. J Am Dent Assoc 2004;135:1413-1426.

Bader JD, Shugars DA, Bonito AJ: A systematic review of selected caries prevention and management methods. Community Dent Oral Epidemiol 2001;29:399-411.

Bamzahim M, Shi XQ, Angmar-Månsson B: Secondary caries detection by DIAGNOdent and radiography: A comparative in vitro study. Acta Odontol Scand 2004;62:61-64.

Baseren NM, Gokalp S: Validity of a laser fluorescence system (DIAGNOdent) for detection of occlusal caries in third molars: An in vitro study. J Oral Rehabil 2003;30:1190-1194.

Batwa M, Bergström J, Batwa S, Al-Otaibi M. The effectiveness of chewing stick Miswak on plaque removal. Saudi Dent J 2006; 18: 125-133.

Benson PE, Parkin N, Millett DT, Dyer FE, Vine S, Shah A: Fluorides for the prevention of white spots on teeth during fixed brace treatment. Cochrane Database Syst Rev 2004:CD003809.

Boersma JG, van der Veen MH, Lagerweij MD, Bokhout B, Prahl-Andersen B: Caries prevalence measured with QLF after treatment with fixed orthodontic appliances: Influencing factors. Caries Res 2005;39:41-47.

Boghani C. Morbidity pattern of dental health problems. J Ind Dent Assoc 1978; 50:277-281.

Bratthall D, Hänsel-Petersson G, Sundberg H: Reasons for the caries decline: What do the experts believe? Eur J Oral Sci 1996;104:416-422; discussion 423-415, 430-412.

Carl W, Zambon JJ: Dental health of the rendille and samburu of the northern frontier district of Kenya. N Y State Dent J 1993;59:35-39.

Cortes DF, Ellwood RP, Ekstrand KR: An in vitro comparison of a combined FOTI/visual examination of occlusal caries with other caries diagnostic methods and the effect of stain on their diagnostic performance. Caries Res 2003;37:8-16.

Costa AM, Yamaguti PM, De Paula LM, Bezerra AC: In vitro study of laser diode 655 nm diagnosis of occlusal caries. ASDC J Dent Child 2002;69:249-253, 233.

Danielsen B, Baelum V, Manji F, Fejerskov O: Chewing sticks, toothpaste, and plaque removal. Acta Odontol Scand 1989;47:121-125.

Darout IA, Albandar JM, Skaug N: Periodontal status of adult Sudanese habitual users of miswak chewing sticks or toothbrushes. Acta Odontol Scand 2000;58:25-30.

Derks A, Katsaros C, Frencken JE, van't Hof MA, Kuijpers-Jagtman AM: Caries-inhibiting effect of preventive measures during orthodontic treatment with fixed appliances. A systematic review. Caries Res 2004;38:413-420.

Eid MA, Selim HA: A retrospective study on the relationship between miswak chewing stick and periodontal health. Egypt Dent J 1994;40:589-592.

Ellwood R, Fejerskov O, Cury JA, Clarkson B. Fluorides in caries control. In: Fejerskov O, Kidd E, editors. Dental caries. The disease and its clinical management. 2nd ed. Oxford, UK; Blackwell Munksgaard 2008:287-327.

Elvin-Lewis M. Plants used for teeth cleaning throughout the World. J Prev Dent 1980;6:61±70.

Elvin-Lewis M: The therapeutic potential of plants used in dental folk medicine. Odontostomatol Trop 1982;5:107-117.

Elvin-Lewis M, Hall JB, Adu-Tuta M, Afful Y, Asante-Appiah K, Lieberman D. The dental health of chewing-stick users of Southern Ghana: Preliminary findings. J Prev Dent 1980; 6: 151-159.

Ezmirly ST, Cheng JC, Wilson SR: Saudi Arabian medicinal plants: Salvadora persica. Planta Med 1979;35:191-192.

Featherstone JD: Prevention and reversal of dental caries: Role of low level fluoride. Community Dent Oral Epidemiol 1999;27:31-40.

Featherstone JD: The science and practice of caries prevention. J Am Dent Assoc 2000;131:887-899.

Fejerskov O, Nyvad B, Kidd EAM: Clinical and histological manifestations of dental caries. In: Fejerskov O, Kidd EAM, eds. Dental caries. The disease and its clinical management, 3d edn. Copenhagen: Blackwell Munksgaard 2003:71-97.

Francescut P, Lussi A: Correlation between fissure discoloration, DIAGNOdent measurements, and caries depth: An in vitro study. Pediatr Dent 2003;25:559-564.

Fung L, Smales R, Ngo H, Moun G: Diagnostic comparison of three groups of examiners using visual and laser fluorescence methods to detect occlusal caries in vitro. Aust Dent J 2004;49:67-71; quiz 101.

Fure S, Gahnberg L, Birkhed D: A comparison of four home-care fluoride programs on the caries incidence in the elderly. Gerodontology 1998;15:51-60.

Gandeh MB, Milaat WA: Dental caries among schoolchildren: Report of a health education campaign in Jeddah, Saudi Arabia. East Mediterr Health J 2000;6:396-401.

Gazi MI, Davies TJ, al-Bagieh N, Cox SW: The immediate- and medium-term effects of Meswak on the composition of mixed saliva. J Clin Periodontol 1992;19:113-117.

Gerrit B. The Miswak, an aspect of dental care in Islam. Medical History 1993; 37: 68-79.

Gorelick L, Geiger AM, Gwinnett AJ: Incidence of white spot formation after bonding and banding. Am J Orthod 1982;81:93-98.

Gorton J, Featherstone JD: In vivo inhibition of demineralization around orthodontic brackets. Am J Orthod Dentofacial Orthop 2003;123:10-14.

Granath LE, Rootzen H, Liljegren E, Holst K, Köhler L: Variation in caries prevalence related to combinations of dietary and oral hygiene habits and chewing fluoride tablets in 4-year-old children. Caries Res 1978;12:83-92.

Grant J: Miswak--toothbrushes that grow on trees. Todays FDA 1990;2:6D.

Hardie J, Ahmed K: The miswak as an aid in oral hygiene. FDI World 1995a;4:5-8, 10.

Hardie J, Ahmed K: The miswak as an aid in oral hygiene. J Philipp Dent Assoc 1995b;47:33-38.

Hattab FN: Meswak: The natural toothbrush. J Clin Dent 1997;8:125-129.

Ismail AI: Visual and visuo-tactile detection of dental caries. J Dent Res 2004;83 Spec No C:C56-66.

Ismail AI, Sohn W, Tellez M, Amaya A, Sen A, Hasson H, Pitts NB: The International caries Detection and Assessment System (ICDAS): An integrated system for measuring dental caries. Community Dent Oral Epidemiol 2007;35:170-178.

Kashani H: Studies on fluoridated toothpicks. Swed Dent J Suppl 1998;126:1-48.

Kashani H, Birkhed D, Petersson LG: Uptake and release of fluoride from birch and lime toothpicks. Eur J Oral Sci 1995;103:112-115.

Kashani H, Birkhed D, Petersson LG: Fluoride concentration in the approximal area after using toothpicks and other fluoride-containing products. Eur J Oral Sci 1998a;106:564-570.

Kashani H, Emilson CG, Birkhed D: Effect of NaF-, SnF2-, and chlorhexidine-impregnated birch toothpicks on mutans streptococci and ph in approximal dental plaque. Acta Odontol Scand 1998b;56:197-201.

Khoory T: The use of chewing sticks in preventive oral hygiene. Clin Prev Dent 1983;5:11-14.

Ko AC, Hewko M, Sowa MG, Dong CC, Cleghorn B, Choo-Smith LP: Early dental caries detection using a fibre-optic coupled polarization-resolved Raman spectroscopic system. Opt Express 2008;16:6274-6284.

Kordic A, Lussi A, Luder HU: Performance of visual inspection, electrical conductance and laser fluorescence in detecting occlusal caries in vitro. Schweiz Monatsschr Zahnmed 2003;113:852-859.

Li J, Nakagaki H, Tsuboi S, Kato S, Huang S, Mukai M, Robinson C, Strong M: Fluoride profiles in different surfaces of human permanent molar enamels from a naturally fluoridated and a non-fluoridated area. Arch Oral Biol 1994;39:727-731.

Lingström P, Holm AK, Mejàre I, Twetman S, Söder B, Norlund A, Axelsson S, Lagerlöf F, Nordenram G, Petersson LG, Dahlgren H, Källestål C: Dietary factors in the prevention of dental caries: A systematic review. Acta Odontol Scand 2003;61:331-340.

Lovrov S, Hertrich K, Hirschfelder U: Enamel demineralization during fixed orthodontic treatment - incidence and correlation to various oral-hygiene parameters. J Orofac Orthop 2007;68:353-363.

Lussi A, Imwinkelried S, Pitts N, Longbottom C, Reich E: Performance and reproducibility of a laser fluorescence system for detection of occlusal caries in vitro. Caries Res 1999;33:261-266.

Lussi A, Megert B, Longbottom C, Reich E, Francescut P: Clinical performance of a laser fluorescence device for detection of occlusal caries lesions. Eur J Oral Sci 2001;109:14-19.

Marinho VC, Higgins JP, Logan S, Sheiham A: Fluoride mouthrinses for preventing dental caries in children and adolescents. Cochrane Database Syst Rev 2003a:CD002284.

Marinho VC, Higgins JP, Logan S, Sheiham A: Topical fluoride (toothpastes, mouthrinses, gels or varnishes) for preventing dental caries in children and adolescents. Cochrane Database Syst Rev 2003b:CD002782.

Marinho VC, Higgins JP, Sheiham A, Logan S: Fluoride toothpastes for preventing dental caries in children and adolescents. Cochrane Database Syst Rev 2003c:CD002278.

Marinho VC, Higgins JP, Sheiham A, Logan S: One topical fluoride (toothpastes, or mouthrinses, or gels, or varnishes) versus another for preventing dental caries in children and adolescents. Cochrane Database Syst Rev 2004a:CD002780.

Marinho VC, Higgins JP, Sheiham A, Logan S: Combinations of topical fluoride (toothpastes, mouthrinses, gels, varnishes) versus single topical fluoride for preventing dental caries in children and adolescents. Cochrane Database Syst Rev 2004b:CD002781.

Marsh PD: Microbiologic aspects of dental plaque and dental caries. Dent Clin North Am 1999;43:599-614, v-vi.

Marsh PD, Nyvad B: The oral microflora and biofilms in teeth. In: Fejerskov O, Kidd EAM, eds. Dental caries. The disease and its clinical management, 3d edn. Copenhagen: Blackwell Munksgaard 2003:29-48.

Mejàre I, Lingström P, Petersson LG, Holm AK, Twetman S, Källestål C, Nordenram G, Lagerlöf F, Söder B, Norlund A, Axelsson S, Dahlgren H: Caries-preventive effect of fissure sealants: A systematic review. Acta Odontol Scand 2003;61:321-330.

Mendes FM, Siqueira WL, Mazzitelli JF, Pinheiro SL, Bengtson AL: Performance of DIAGNOdent for detection and quantification of smooth-surface caries in primary teeth. J Dent 2005;33:79-84.

Moberg Sköld U, Birkhed D, Borg E, Petersson LG: Approximal caries development in adolescents with low to moderate caries risk after different 3-year school-based supervised fluoride mouth rinsing programmes. Caries Res 2005;39:529-535.

Mohammad AR, Turner JE: In vitro evaluation of Saudi Arabian toothbrush tree (Salvadora persica). Odontostomatol Trop 1983;6:145-148.

Mørch T, Bjørvatn K: Laboratory study of fluoride impregnated toothpicks. Scand J Dent Res 1981;89:499-505.

Ng'ang'a PM, Øgaard B: Dental caries and fluorides in relation to fixed orthodontic treatment: A review. East Afr Med J 1993;70:75-77.

Norton MR, Addy M: Chewing sticks versus toothbrushes in West Africa. A pilot study. Clin Prev Dent 1989;11:11-13.

Øgaard B: Prevalence of white spot lesions in 19-year-olds: A study on untreated and orthodontically treated persons 5 years after treatment. Am J Orthod Dentofacial Orthop 1989a;96:423-427.

Øgaard B: [Cariologic aspects of orthodontic treatment]. Nor Tannlaegeforen Tid 1989b;99:802-805.

Øgaard B, Rølla G, Arends J: Orthodontic appliances and enamel demineralization. Part 1. Lesion development. Am J Orthod Dentofacial Orthop 1988;94:68-73.

Øgaard B, Seppä L, Rølla G: Professional topical fluoride applications--clinical efficacy and mechanism of action. Adv Dent Res 1994;8:190-201.

Ouellet A, Hondrum SO, Pietz DM: Detection of occlusal carious lesions. Gen Dent 2002;50:346-350.

Penick C: Power toothbrushes: A critical review. Int J Dent Hyg 2004;2:40-44.

Petersen PE, Mzee MO: Oral health profile of schoolchildren, mothers and schoolteachers in Zanzibar. Community Dent Health 1998;15:256-262.

Petersson LG, Kashani H, Birkhed D: In vitro and in vivo studies of an NaF impregnated toothpick. Swed Dent J 1994;18:69-73.

Pitts N: "ICDAS"--an international system for caries detection and assessment being developed to facilitate caries epidemiology, research and appropriate clinical management. Community Dent Health 2004;21:193-198.

Rølla G, Ekstrand J. Fluoride in oral fluids and dental plaque. In: Fluoride in dentistry. Eds, Fejerskov O, Ekstrand J, Burt BA. Munksgaard 1996:215-229.

Särner B, Birkhed D, Lingström P: Approximal fluoride concentration using different fluoridated products alone or in combination. Caries Res 2008;42:73-78.

Särner B, Lingström P, Birkhed D: Fluoride release from NaF- and AmF-impregnated toothpicks and dental flosses in vitro and in vivo. Acta Odontol Scand 2003;61:289-296.

Sathananthan K, Vos T, Bango G: Dental caries, fluoride levels and oral hygiene practices of school children in Matabeleland South, Zimbabwe. Community Dent Oral Epidemiol 1996;24:21-24.

SBU. Att förebygga karies. En systematisk litteraturöversikt. Rapport 161, Elanders Graphic Systems, 2002 (in Swedish).

Schier M, Cleaton-Jones P: Dental caries in Namibia--the first national survey. Community Dent Oral Epidemiol 1995;23:262-265.

Selwitz RH, Ismail AI, Pitts NB: Dental caries. Lancet 2007;369:51-59.

Shi XQ, Welander U, Angmar-Månsson B: Occlusal caries detection with kavo DIAGNOdent and radiography: An in vitro comparison. Caries Res 2000;34:151-158.

Sköld-Larsson K, Fornell AC, Lussi A, Twetman S: Effect of topical applications of a chlorhexidine/thymol-containing varnish on fissure caries assessed by laser fluorescence. Acta Odontol Scand 2004;62:339-342.

Sofrata A, Lingström P, Baljoon M, Gustafsson A: The effect of miswak extract on plaque pH. An in vivo study. Caries Res 2007;41:451-454.

Sofrata AH, Claesson RL, Lingström PK, Gustafsson AK: Strong antibacterial effect of miswak against oral microorganisms associated with periodontitis and caries. J Periodontol 2008;79:1474-1479.

Staudt CB, Lussi A, Jacquet J, Kiliaridis S: White spot lesions around brackets: In vitro detection by laser fluorescence. Eur J Oral Sci 2004;112:237-243.

Stoodley P, Wefel J, Gieseke A, Debeer D, von Ohle C: Biofilm plaque and hydrodynamic effects on mass transfer, fluoride delivery and caries. J Am Dent Assoc 2008;139:1182-1190.

Sudjalim TR, Woods MG, Manton DJ: Prevention of white spot lesions in orthodontic practice: A contemporary review. Aust Dent J 2006;51:284-289; quiz 347.

Sudjalim TR, Woods MG, Manton DJ, Reynolds EC: Prevention of demineralization around orthodontic brackets in vitro. Am J Orthod Dentofacial Orthop 2007;131:705 e701-709.

ten Cate JM: Review on fluoride, with special emphasis on calcium fluoride mechanisms in caries prevention. Eur J Oral Sci 1997;105:461-465.

ten Cate JM: Current concepts on the theories of the mechanism of action of fluoride. Acta Odontol Scand 1999;57:325-329.

ten Cate JM, Buijs MJ, Miller CC, Exterkate RA: Elevated fluoride products enhance remineralization of advanced enamel lesions. J Dent Res 2008;87:943-947.

ten Cate JM, Damen JJ, Buijs MJ: Inhibition of dentin demineralization by fluoride in vitro. Caries Res 1998;32:141-147.

Twetman S, Axelsson S, Dahlgren H, Holm AK, Källestål C, Lagerlöf F, Lingström P, Mejàre I, Nordenram G, Norlund A, Petersson LG, Söder B: Caries-preventive effect of fluoride toothpaste: A systematic review. Acta Odontol Scand 2003;61:347-355.

Twetman S, Petersson L, Axelsson S, Dahlgren H, Holm AK, Källestål C, Lagerlöf F, Lingström P, Mejàre I, Nordenram G, Norlund A, Söder B: Caries-preventive effect of sodium fluoride mouthrinses: A systematic review of controlled clinical trials. Acta Odontol Scand 2004;62:223-230.

Villa A, Anabalon M, Zohouri V, Maguire A, Franco AM, Rugg-Gunn A: Relationships between fluoride intake, urinary fluoride excretion and fluoride retention in children and adults: An analysis of available data. Caries Res;44:60-68.

WHO: Preventive methods and programmes for oral diseases. World Health Organization. Technical Report Series 713, Geneva;1987.

Wiegand A, Buchalla W, Attin T: Review on fluoride-releasing restorative materials--fluoride release and uptake characteristics, antibacterial activity and influence on caries formation. Dent Mater 2007;23:343-362.

Wu CD, Darout IA, Skaug N: Chewing sticks: Timeless natural toothbrushes for oral cleansing. J Periodontal Res 2001;36:275-284.

Wyne A, Al-Dlaigan Y, Khan N: Caries prevalence, oral hygiene and orthodontic status of Saudi Bedouin children. Indian J Dent Res 2001;12:194-198.

Zimmer S: Caries-preventive effects of fluoride products when used in conjunction with fluoride dentifrice. Caries Res 2001;35 Suppl 1:18-21.

I

Original Paper

Caries Research

Caries Res 2008;42:363–368
DOI: 10.1159/000151588

Received: March 5, 2008
Accepted after revision: June 30, 2008
Published online: August 27, 2008

Uptake and Release of Fluoride from Fluoride-Impregnated Chewing Sticks (Miswaks) in vitro and in vivo

H.A. Baeshen[a, b]   H. Kjellberg[b]   P. Lingström[a, c]   D. Birkhed[a]

Departments of [a]Cariology and [b]Orthodontics, Sahlgrenska Academy at University of Gothenburg, Gothenburg, and [c]Department of Health Sciences, Kristianstad University, Kristianstad, Sweden

Key Words

Approximal area · Chewing stick (miswak) · Fluoride impregnation · Saliva

To conclude, NaF-impregnated miswaks produced a rapid release of F in vitro as well as in vivo and may be an interesting vehicle for home care use for caries prevention in countries where they are used regularly.

Abstract

The purpose was to investigate the uptake and release of fluoride (F) from F-impregnated chewing sticks (miswaks). In the first series, 3-cm-long pieces were impregnated in 1, 2, 3 and 4% NaF solutions for 3 h, 1 day and 3 days (10 pieces/test). There was a dose-response effect with respect to both impregnation time and the concentration of the F solution. In the second and third series, totally 40 miswak pieces were impregnated in 3% NaF for 1 day and 3 days; the outer layer (bark) was separated from the inner spongy part (pulp) and analyzed separately. F was released from both parts, but somewhat more was released from the bark than from the pulp; a plateau was reached at around 30 min. In vivo, 9 healthy subjects used three products for 2 min in a crossover design: (1) a miswak impregnated in 3% NaF for 1 day, (2) a miswak impregnated in 3% NaF for 3 days, and (3) 1 g of F toothpaste (containing 1,450 ppm F as NaF) on a toothbrush. The highest F concentration at the approximal area was obtained after using the miswak impregnated in 3% NaF for 3 days compared with the other products ($p < 0.05$ or $p < 0.01$).

Methods for oral hygiene vary from one country to the other as well as among cultures. Despite the widespread use of toothbrushes and toothpastes, tooth cleaning with chewing sticks (in Arabic *miswak*, 'a tooth-cleaning stick' [Hattab, 1997]), prepared from twigs, stems or roots, which has been practiced for thousands of years in Asia, Africa, the Middle East and United States, is still in use [Darout et al., 2002; Al-Otaibi et al., 2004]. In some parts of the world, particularly in rural areas, the use of miswaks is common [Asadi et al., 1997; Petersen and Mzee, 1998] and the World Health Organization has recommended and encouraged the use of chewing sticks as an effective tool for oral hygiene [World Health Organization, 1987]. Data from 6 Saudi Arabian regions indicate that 3/4 of males and 2/3 of females use a miswak regularly [Almas et al., 2000]. Among urban Saudi Arabians, more than 70% used a toothbrush, while a miswak was used daily by more than 60%, with varia-

KARGER

Fax +41 61 306 12 34
E-Mail karger@karger.ch
www.karger.com

© 2008 S. Karger AG, Basel
0008–6568/08/0425–0363$24.50/0

Accessible online at:
www.karger.com/cre

Dowen Birkhed
Department of Cariology
Institute of Odontology, Box 450
SE–405 30 Göteborg (Sweden)
Tel. +46 31 786 3201, Fax +46 31 825 733, E-Mail birkhed@odontologi.gu.se

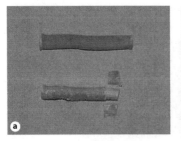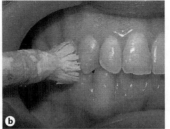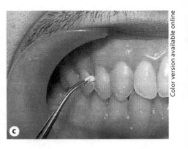

Fig. 1. a A miswak both with and without the outer layer (bark). **b** The use of a miswak for cleaning the teeth. **c** Sampling of approximal saliva.

tions in relation to age, gender and socioeconomic background [Al-Otaibi et al., 2003].

Miswaks are harvested from the plant *Salvadora persica,* which grows in the Middle East, in some Asian countries and in Africa [Almas, 2001]. Miswaks were originally used for cleaning purposes only. However, several studies have shown an antimicrobial effect, both with respect to dental caries and to periodontal disease [Almas, 2001; Darout et al., 2002, 2003; Almas and Al-Zeid, 2004].

A large number of home care fluoride (F) products, such as toothpaste, rinsing solutions, tablets and chewing gums, are found on the market today. In the early 1980s, the idea of impregnating wooden toothpicks with F was first described by Mörch and Bjorvatn [1981]. Nowadays, not only F toothpicks, but also fluoridated dental flosses are available in Europe and the USA [Kashani et al., 1998; Särner et al., 2003, 2005].

Since miswaks do not naturally contain F [Wu et al., 2001] and are rather porous (and thus suitable for impregnation), we thought it would be of interest to fluoridate this type of product. Therefore, the aim of the present investigation was to study the uptake and release of F from F-impregnated miswaks both in vitro and in vivo.

Materials and Methods

Fresh miswaks were brought from the Kingdom of Saudi Arabia, transported to Sweden and kept in a refrigerator for 2 weeks before use. The miswaks were cut with a scalpel into 3-cm-long pieces. Before impregnation, they were kept in distilled water for 6 h and then dried in an oven (40°C) overnight (approx. 12 h) and weighed using an electronic balance. The miswaks were then impregnated in NaF. After impregnation, they were removed from the solution by a forceps and placed on paper at room temperature overnight (approx. 12 h) in order to dry; they were then weighed again. The difference in weight of each miswak before and after impregnation was calculated in order to measure the uptake of NaF.

In some series, the outer layer (bark) was peeled off from the inner spongy part (pulp) and analyzed separately (fig. 1a).

One nonimpregnated miswak and one impregnated with 3% NaF were air-dried, sputter-coated with gold and examined using a scanning electron microscope (SEM; Leica S420; Leica Microsystems Heidelberg, Germany), equipped with LEO Software 15XX).

In vitro Studies

Three series were carried out. In the first, 120 miswak pieces (10 pieces × 4 concentrations × 3 time points) were impregnated in 1, 2, 3 and 4% NaF solutions for 3 h, 1 day and 3 days. In the second series, 20 miswaks were impregnated in 3% NaF for 1 day only. The bark was separated from the pulp and placed in a separate vial. The third series was identical to the second, except that the impregnation time was prolonged to 3 days.

The miswaks were placed in 150 ml NaF solution in a 250-ml glass bottle. After impregnation, each individual piece of miswak was placed on paper and air-dried overnight (approx. 12 h). After drying, they were transferred to a plastic 20-ml bottle with 15 ml of distilled water and 1.5 ml TISAB III solution (Orion Research, Boston, Mass., USA). Aliquots of 0.3 ml were taken with a pipette at 0, 1, 2, 5, 10, 15, 30, 40, and 60 min, transferred to a 2-ml plastic beaker covered with a lid and kept in a refrigerator for up to 1 week before the F analysis.

In vivo Studies

Nine healthy adult subjects, mean age 60 years, were selected among the staff at the University of Göteborg. Three different fluoridated products were tested: (1) miswak impregnated in 3% NaF for 1 day, (2) miswak impregnated in 3% NaF for 3 days, and (3) 1 g of F toothpaste (containing 1,450 ppm F as NaF) applied on a toothbrush. The three products were tested in a randomized order. The bark of the miswak was first removed as in ordinary use (fig. 1a). It was then chewed for a short time (3–5 s) and moved around the dentition for cleaning all buccal and buccally oriented approximal surfaces during 2 min (fig. 1b). Toothbrushing with F toothpaste was carried out in a normal manner for 2 min.

Table 1. The accumulated release of F (in ppm) from miswaks in vitro during 60 min when impregnated in 1, 2, 3 or 4% NaF for 3 h, 1 day and 3 days

	Impreg-nation	Accumulated release of F				
		1 min	5 min	15 min	30 min	60 min
3 h	1%	0.7 ± 0.6	1.0 ± 1.1	3.6 ± 3.0	5.6 ± 2.8	11.0 ± 3.5
	2%	0.9 ± 0.9	3.9 ± 2.9	6.4 ± 3.3	12.2 ± 5.0	18.4 ± 5.8
	3%	0.8 ± 0.7	3.0 ± 2.6	6.9 ± 3.8	12.6 ± 7.2	21.0 ± 7.2
	4%	3.7 ± 3.4	15.9 ± 8.2	34.3 ± 14.3	33.5 ± 16.0	42.4 ± 15.4
1 day	1%	1.1 ± 1.1	4.4 ± 4.0	9.1 ± 4.7	16.6 ± 5.3	17.0 ± 4.0
	2%	0.6 ± 0.5	3.5 ± 4.1	5.1 ± 4.5	15.4 ± 9.8	18.6 ± 10.7
	3%	2.3 ± 2.7	5.3 ± 9.0	13.7 ± 20.1	22.8 ± 32.3	30.2 ± 31.1
	4%	13.6 ± 34.6	21.8 ± 41.0	56.2 ± 74.0	63.0 ± 76.2	96.0 ± 122.7
3 days	1%	1.7 ± 2.9	2.6 ± 4.5	12.1 ± 8.4	12.6 ± 6.7	17.5 ± 5.8
	2%	2.7 ± 4.5	33.1 ± 57.8	71.3 ± 83.0	92.7 ± 102.3	121.8 ± 82.9
	3%	42.7 ± 47.6	115.2 ± 62.5	262.3 ± 147.1	321.8 ± 178.0	384.8 ± 169.5
	4%	87.6 ± 140.9	505.2 ± 376.4	705.8 ± 271.2	789.8 ± 224.6	836.2 ± 314.5

Mean values ± SD of 10 samples/test.

Sampling of two approximal sites (14/15 and 24/25) was carried out before (0 min; baseline) and 1, 3, 5, 7, 9, 15 and 30 min after finishing the 2-min cleaning procedure. Small triangle-shaped paper points (base: 1.5 mm; length: 5 mm) were inserted in the approximal area for 30 s in order to suck up around 4 μl of saliva (fig. 1c) [Kashani et al., 1998].

Analysis of Fluoride

The F concentration was determined by means of an F-sensitive electrode connected to an ion analyzer (Orion Research). Ionic strength was stabilized by adding TISAB III according to the manufacturer's instructions (in the F release experiments, TISAB had been added to the solution into which the release occurred and no further addition was required). All analyses were performed using standard solutions from 0.526 μM (0.01 ppm) to 5.26 mM (100 ppm) F. The detection limit of F was approximately 0.5 μM.

For the in vivo study, each paper point was transferred to a 0.5-ml Eppendorf tube, containing 200 μl distilled water and 20 μl TISAB III (Orion Research). The absorbed F was allowed to diffuse from the paper point into the solution for 24 h in the refrigerator. Prior to analysis, the samples were thoroughly mixed by vibration for 10 s. The F concentration was then analyzed using the ion-specific electrode.

Statistical Method

The area under the curve (AUC) was calculated for each individual and each treatment. Statistical comparisons were made using two-way analysis of variance, followed by a multiple comparison test with Fisher's protected least significant difference to compare the AUC values for different procedures in vivo; $p < 0.05$ was considered statistically significant.

Results

In vitro Studies

No F was found in the nonimpregnated miswaks (data not shown). F release from miswaks after 1, 5, 15, 30 and 60 min under the various conditions is shown in table 1. The higher the NaF concentration used and the longer the impregnation time, the more release of F was found. There were large standard deviations. A clear dose-response effect with respect to F concentration and impregnation time was found. The release was approximately constant with time, after a period of rapid release during the first 10 min, especially after impregnation in 3 and 4% NaF for 3 days (fig. 2).

The release of F from the bark and pulp impregnated in 3% NaF for 3 days is shown in figure 3. The bark released more F than the pulp, but both parts gave high and fast release, especially during the first 10 min. Miswaks impregnated in 3% NaF for 1 day showed a similar pattern (data not shown).

The differences in weight of dried miswaks before and after 3 h of impregnation with NaF solution showed that the higher the NaF concentration used, the more the uptake of F by the miswak (table 2).

In SEM images of a miswak impregnated in 3% NaF there were snow flake-like crystals on the outer layer (fig. 4). However, the shape of these crystals appeared different from those of NaF crystals formed on glass (not shown).

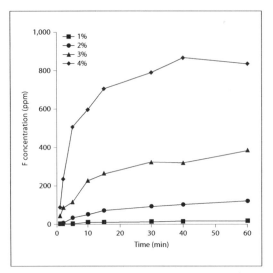

Fig. 2. The release of F in vitro from miswaks during 60 min. Each miswak was impregnated in 1, 2, 3 or 4% NaF for 3 days, dried and placed in 5 ml distilled water (mean values of 10 samples/test).

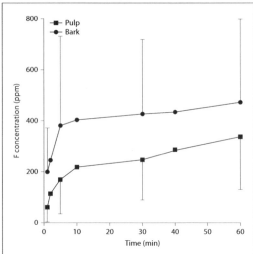

Fig. 3. The release of F from the bark and the pulp of a miswak impregnated in 3% NaF for 3 days (mean values of 20 samples/test). The standard deviation is only given in one direction and only for every second value.

In vivo Studies

Figure 5 shows the F concentration and AUC values in the approximal area after using fluoridated miswaks and F toothpaste. The F concentration was elevated during the whole 30-min period. The AUC was twice as high for the miswak impregnated for 3 days than for that impregnated for 1 day and 4 times higher than for F toothpaste ($p < 0.05$ and $p < 0.01$, respectively).

Discussion

The data from the present study clearly show that both the uptake and release of F from impregnated miswaks are fast processes. The quick release may be explained by the fact that wood can absorb and retain NaF solution both on the surface (bark) and in porosities of the inner spongy part (pulp). SEM studies confirmed this statement. The reason why the NaF crystals looked different on the miswak than on glass may depend on the reaction with miswak components. The uptake and release of F depend on several factors, such as the porosity, the size and the nature of a miswak. Cross sections of miswak show that the plants are indeed very spongy [Al-Otaibi,

Table 2. Weight (in g) after drying of 3-cm-long miswaks before and after impregnation in NaF solution for 3 h

	Before impregnation	After impregnation	Difference (uptake)
NaF concentration			
1%	1.20 ± 0.18	1.41 ± 0.15	0.20 ± 0.04
2%	1.19 ± 0.12	1.42 ± 0.12	0.24 ± 0.03
3%	1.19 ± 0.12	1.61 ± 0.16	0.42 ± 0.11
4%	1.18 ± 0.10	1.65 ± 0.12	0.47 ± 0.06

The difference indicates the uptake of NaF (mean values ± SD of 10 pieces/test).

2004]. All these factors may influence retention of NaF, which easily redissolves on contact with a liquid such as saliva. It is therefore an advantage to moisten the fluoridated miswaks in the mouth for a few seconds just before they are used in order to speed up the F release process.

In vitro, the F release showed a clear dose-response effect with respect to both F concentration and impregnation time. Thus, the higher concentration in the impregnating solution, the more F was absorbed, resulting in a

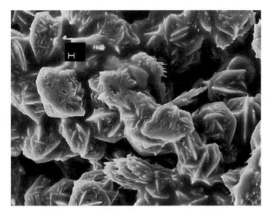

Fig. 4. SEM of the outer surface (bark) of a miswak impregnated in 3% NaF for 1 day.

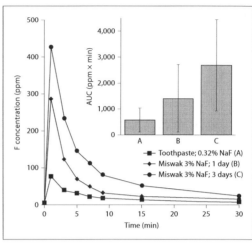

Fig. 5. F concentration in approximal saliva in vivo after brushing with 1 g of 0.32% NaF toothpaste (A), using a miswak impregnated in 3% NaF for 1 day (B) and using a miswak impregnated in 3% NaF for 3 days (C) (mean values of 9 individuals). The bars show the AUC values and SD for each treatment.

higher release from the miswak. These results are in agreement with studies on fluoridated wooden toothpicks [Kashani et al., 1995]. In vivo, more F was released into saliva when the miswak was impregnated in 3% NaF for 3 days compared to 1 day. The F release from the bark of the miswak was higher than from the pulp. This could be due to the fact that the outer layer is thin and more porous than the inner spongy part. Still, F can reach the pulp which, after peeling off the outer layer, is used for cleaning the teeth.

When using a fluoridated miswak, a relatively large surface area of the pulp of the chewing stick will come in contact with saliva. This means that F is released into the oral cavity and subsequently swallowed. In the in vivo experiments, miswaks impregnated with 3% NaF for 3 days gave, when calculated as AUC, about 5 times more F in the oral cavity than the 0.32% NaF toothpaste. It has to be remembered that all of this F from the miswak will be swallowed in contrast to F from toothpaste. Therefore, before fluoridated miswaks are introduced on the market, it is important that the fluoridation procedure is standardized and that the product is launched under controlled conditions. This is of special importance since miswaks may be used up to 5–6 times a day.

Miswaks are commonly used in many Arabic countries, such as Saudi Arabia, known to have a high prevalence of dental caries [Al Dosari et al., 2004]. Every time a miswak is used, the used part is cut off and a new fresh part is peeled and used. Therefore, we believe that it is interesting from a caries prevention point of view to in-

troduce fluoridated miswaks on a large scale in these countries. This is of special interest because miswaks are used prior to each prayer, which means several times every day. Some individuals even use the miswaks after eating, which may be favorable for prevention of dental caries.

In conclusion, NaF-impregnated miswaks showed a quick release of F both in vitro and in vivo. We therefore believe that this type of chewing stick is an interesting F vehicle in those countries where they are used commonly. Further studies on fluoridated miswaks should be carried out in order to evaluate the clinical effect and to optimize the fluoridation procedure.

Acknowledgements

We thank Ann-Britt Lundberg, Department of Cariology, for her technical support, Elena Linder, Department of Periodontology, for the scanning electron microscopy, and Dr. Meshari Al-Otaibi, Kingdom of Saudi Arabia, for introducing us into research on miswaks.

References

Al Dosari AM, Wyne AH, Akpata ES, Khan NB: Caries prevalence and its relation to water fluoride levels among schoolchildren in central province of Saudi Arabia. Int Dent J 2004;54:424–428.

Almas K: The antimicrobial effects of seven different types of Asian chewing sticks. Trop Dent J 2001;24:17–20.

Almas K, Albaker A, Felemban N: Knowledge of dental health and diseases among dental patients, a multicenter study in Saudi Arabia. Indian J Dent Res 2000;11:145–155.

Almas K, Al-Zeid Z: The immediate antimicrobial effect of a toothbrush and Miswak on cariogenic bacteria: a clinical study. J Contemp Dent Pract 2004;5:105–114.

Al-Otaibi M: The Miswak (chewing stick) and oral health. Studies on oral hygiene practices of urban Saudi Arabia. Swed Dent J Suppl 2004;167:2–75.

Al-Otaibi M, Al-Harthy M, Gustafsson A, Johansson A, Claesson R, Angmar-Månsson B: Subgingival plaque microbiota in Saudi Arabians after use of Miswak chewing stick and toothbrush. J Clin Periodontol 2004;31:1048–1053.

Al-Otaibi M, Zimmerman M, Angmar-Månsson B: Prevailing oral hygiene practices among urban Saudi Arabians in relation to age, gender and socio-economic background. Acta Odontol Scand 2003;61:212–216.

Asadi SGR, Asadi ZG: Chewing sticks and the oral hygiene habits of adult Pakistani population. Int Dent J 1997;47:275–278.

Darout IA, Albandar JM, Skaug N, Ali RW: Salivary microbiota levels in relation to periodontal status, experience of caries and miswak use in Sudanese adults. J Clin Periodontol 2002;29:411–420.

Darout IA, Skuag N, Albandar JM: Subgingival microbiota levels and their associations with periodontal status at the sampled sites in an adult Sudanese population using Miswak or toothbrush regularly. Acta Odontol Scand 2003;61:115–122.

Hattab FN: Miswak: the natural toothbrush. J Clin Dent 1997;8:125–129.

Kashani H, Birkhed D, Petersson LG: Uptake and release of fluoride from birch and lime toothpicks. Eur J Oral Sci 1995;103:112–115.

Kashani H, Birkhed D, Petersson LG: Fluoride concentration in the approximal area after using toothpicks and other fluoride-containing products. Eur J Oral Sci 1998;106:564–570.

Mörch T, Bjørvatn K: Laboratory study of fluoride impregnated toothpicks. Scand J Dent Res 1981;89:499–505.

Petersen PE, Mzee MO: Oral health profile of schoolchildren, mothers and school teachers in Zanzibar. Community Dent Health 1998; 15:256–262.

Särner B, Birkhed D, Huysmans MC, Ruben JL, Fidler V, Lingström P: Effect of fluoridated toothpicks and dental flosses on enamel and dentine and on plaque composition in situ. Caries Res 2005;39:52–59.

Särner B, Lingström P, Birkhed D: Fluoride release from NaF- and AmF-impregnated toothpicks and dental flosses in vitro and in vivo. Caries Res 2003;61:289–296.

World Health Organization: Preventive Methods and Programmes for Oral Diseases. Technical Report Series 713. Geneva, World Health Organization, 1987.

Wu CD, Darout IA, Skaug N: Chewing sticks: timeless natural toothbrushes for oral cleansing. J Periodontal Res 2001;36:275–284.

II

Release of Fluoride from Fresh and Old NaF-Impregnated Chewing Sticks (Miswaks) *In Vitro* and Oral Retention *In Vivo*

Hosam Baeshen[a]/Dowen Birkhed[a]

Purpose: The objectives of the present investigation were to study fluoride (F) release from NaF-impregnated chewing sticks (Miswaks) *in vitro* and to study the F clearance in saliva and the F oral retention *in vivo*.

Materials and Methods: Both fresh and old Miswaks were collected from 10 stores in Saudi Arabia and fluoridated in 0.01%, 0.1%, 0.5%, 1% and 3% NaF. The F release was studied *in vitro* up to 60 min. *In vivo*, 10 subjects used Miswaks fluoridated in 0.01%, 0.1%, 0.5%, 1% and 3% NaF for 2 min (Series I). The subjects were asked to spit out all saliva in a beaker during a 12-min period without swallowing. The F present in the obtained saliva was considered to represent the 'F retention'. In Series II, the same type of Miswaks were used as in Series I. Repeated whole saliva unstimulated samples were collected before and up to 30 min after. These two series were carried out in another 10 subjects (Series III and IV), but with Miswaks fluoridated in a more narrow range of concentration (0.05% to 0.5% NaF). Brushing with 1 g of F-containing dentifrice (0.32% NaF) was used as a control.

Results: There were only small differences between fresh and old Miswaks, but great variations were observed between Miswaks that were purchased from different stores. Miswaks fluoridated in 0.1% to 0.5% NaF could be considered as an 'optimum level' with respect to both the F concentration in saliva and the F retention.

Conclusions: It is recommended to use fresh Miswaks impregnated in 0.1% NaF or a maximum of 0.5% NaF for a day, as they are interesting and safe products for the prevention of caries and could be widely used in countries such as Saudi Arabia.

Key words: chewing stick, fluoride, fluoride retention, impregnation, Miswak, saliva, *Salvadora persica*

Oral Health Prev Dent 2010; 8: 93–99.   Submitted for publication: 19.02.09; accepted for publication: 14.10.09.

Nowadays, manual and electric toothbrushes are being used in most industrialised countries, whereas in the developing world these products are still rare (Al-Otaibi et al, 2004). Instead, chewing sticks (Miswaks) made from trees and shrubs are commonly used (Hardie and Ahmed, 1995; Wu et al, 2001; Darout et al, 2002; Al-Otaibi et al, 2004). Miswak is an Arabic word which means 'a tooth-cleaning stick' (Hattab, 1997). It is harvested from the plant *Salvadora persica* (also called 'toothbrush tree'), which grows in the Middle East, Asia and Africa (Almas, 2001; Wu et al, 2001). Miswaks were originally used for cleaning purposes only. However, several studies have shown that they may have a certain antimicrobial effect, with respect to both gingivitis and caries (Almas, 2001; Wu et al, 2001; Darout et al, 2002, 2003; Almas and Al-Zeid, 2004).

In some parts of the world, particularly in rural areas, the use of Miswaks is quite common (Boghani, 1978; Elvin-Lewis et al, 1980; Khoory, 1983; Asadi and Asadi, 1997; Petersen and Mzee, 1998). Data collected from six regions of Saudi Arabia indicate that three-fourths of males and two-thirds of females regularly use a Miswak, that is, several times in a day (Almas et al, 2000). There are great variations

[a] Department of Cariology, Sahlgrenska Academy, University of Gothenburg, Göteborg, Sweden.

Correspondence: Dowen Birkhed, Department of Cariology, Institute of Odontology, Box 450, SE-405 30 Göteborg, Sweden. Tel: +46 31 7863201. Email: birkhed@odontologi.gu.se observed, however, in oral hygiene habits that are mainly related to age and socioeconomic level in this country (Al-Otaibi et al, 2003). The World Health Organization recommends and encourages the use of chewing sticks for oral hygiene (World Health Organization [WHO], 1987).

In the early 1980s, the idea of impregnating wooden toothpicks with NaF was first described by two Norwegian researchers (Mörch and Bjørvatn, 1981). Nowadays, not only fluoride (F) toothpicks, but also fluoridated dental floss are available in Europe and USA (Kashani et al, 1998; Särner et al, 2003, 2005). A pilot study has recently been conducted on NaF-impregnated Miswaks (Baeshen et al, 2008). The results show a rapid release of F in vitro as well as in vivo. As the results are so promising, the present study extends these previous studies to optimise the fluoridation procedure for clinical use on a broad scale. The aims of the present investigation were (i) to study the variations in F release from fresh and old NaF-impregnated Miswaks in vitro and (ii) to study the F clearance in saliva and the 'F retention' when using Miswaks impregnated in various NaF concentrations.

MATERIALS AND METHODS

Miswaks

For the in vitro studies, Miswaks, both fresh and old types, were purchased from 10 different stores in Jeddah (Kingdom of Saudi Arabia). Each bundle contained 15-cm-long sticks from the tree, S. persica. From these bundles, five different sticks were randomly selected and cut into 3-cm-long pieces, giving a total of 100 Miswaks (50 fresh and 50 old). For the in vivo studies, 25 fresh, 50-cm-long sticks were purchased from the same store and cut into 4-cm-long pieces (to facilitate the handling of Miswak by the patient). For both the in vitro and in vivo studies, the total number of Miswaks used was approximately 400. All of them were collected within a week, taken to Sweden and kept in a refrigerator before use. Miswaks are natural products, and there are great variations observed with regard to size, diameter and colour. An attempt was made to control these factors, by a visual inspection, to have all specimens as similar as possible, especially with respect to size and weight. After cutting and coding, they were kept in distilled water for 6 h (to clean them from dust). They were then dried in an oven at 40°C overnight.

Fluoridation procedure

Five different concentrations (0.01%, 0.1%, 0.5%, 1% and 3%) of NaF were used during the in vitro and in vivo experiments. In two of the in vivo series, 0.05%, 0.1%, 0.2%, 0.3%, 0.4% and 0.5% NaF were also used. For each concentration, Miswaks were placed in a vial containing 500 ml of NaF solution for a day, that is, with an excess of solution. After impregnation, the Miswaks were removed from the bottle (by a forceps) and placed on a paper for drying at room temperature overnight.

In vitro studies

Two series (here called I and II) were carried out. In the first (Series I), the aim was to evaluate the variations in the F release between the fresh and old Miswaks, and in the second (Series II), the aim was to study if there were any differences in the F release between the Miswaks that were purchased from various stores. The NaF-impregnated Miswaks were kept in 20-ml plastic bottles containing 15 ml of distilled water and 1.5 ml of TISAB III solution (Orion Research, Boston, MA, USA). Aliquots (0.3 ml) were taken with a pipette at 0, 2, 10, 30 and 60 min, and were transferred to 2-ml plastic beakers that were covered with a lid. The samples were kept in a refrigerator for 1 to 2 days until analysed.

In vivo studies

Four series (here called I, II, III and IV) were carried out with two sets of NaF concentrations as described in Table 1. Twenty healthy adult subjects (mean age 41 years) were selected from among the staff at the University of Gothenburg (10 for Series I and II and 10 for Series III and IV). Five Miswaks, fluoridated in 0.01%, 0.1%, 0.5%, 1% and 3% NaF for a day (Series I), were tested in a randomised order. The aim of the present experiment was to evaluate how much F is expected to be swallowed (here called 'F retention') when using a Miswak. Each subject was instructed not to brush his/her teeth with an F-containing dentifrice on the day of examination and not to eat or drink 2 h before the test. The bark of the Miswak was first peeled off (Fig 1, upper part). The pulp was then chewed for a short duration (to spread the bristles) and moved around the dentition for cleaning all the buccal and available approximal surfaces for 2 min (Fig 1, lower part). The subject

Table 1 The impregnation procedure and the saliva collection procedure for Series I to IV *in vivo*

Series (n = 10)	NaF impregnation solutions (%)	Saliva sampling
I[1]	0.01, 0.1, 0.5, 1 and 3	Continuous collection during 2 + 10 min
II[1]	As in Series I	At 0, 1, 3, 5, 7, 9, 15 and 30 min
III[2]	0.05, 0.1, 0.2, 0.3, 0.4 and 0.5	As in Series I
IV[2]	As in Series III + F-containing dentifrice	As in Series II

[1]The same 10 subjects were included in Series I and II.
[2]The same 10 subjects were included in Series III and IV.

was instructed not to swallow any saliva, but instead was asked to spit in a beaker during this 2-min period and for the next 10 min. After this 12-min period, the patient finally rinsed the mouth with 20 ml of distilled water for 30 s and spit it out in the same beaker.

In the second (Series II), another five Miswaks impregnated as in Series I were used in a randomised order. The aim of the present experiment was to study the F concentration in saliva when using a fluoridated Miswak. Unstimulated saliva sampling was carried out before (0 min; baseline) and at 1, 3, 5, 7, 9, 15 and 30 min after using the Miswak for 2 min.

Series III and IV were identical to Series I and II, except that a more narrow range of NaF concentrations was used (based on the data from the first two series). Thus, Miswaks that were fluoridated in 0.05%, 0.1%, 0.2%, 0.3%, 0.4% and 0.5% NaF for a day were used. Moreover, the subjects brushed with 1 g of F-containing dentifrice (containing 1450 ppm F as NaF) applied on a toothbrush. All of these seven F products (6 + 1) were tested in 10 healthy subjects in a randomised order (Table 1). The present study was approved by the Ethics Committee of the Sahlgrenska Academy at the University of Gothenburg.

Analysis of Fluoride

The samples were analysed blinded regarding subjects and methods. The F concentration was determined using an F-sensitive electrode connected to an ion analyser (Orion Research). TISAB III was added (1:10) according to the manufacturers' instructions for stabilizing the ionic strength. The electrode was calibrated against three standard solutions from 0.526 µM (0.01 ppm) to 5.26 mM (100 ppm) of F. The detection limit of F was about 0.5 µM.

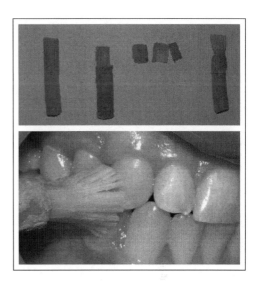

Fig 1 Before use, the bark of the Miswak is peeled off (upper part of the figure). The lower part of the figure shows how the bristles of the pulp come into close contact with the tooth surface when used.

For the *in vivo* studies, 300 µl of each saliva sample in Series II and IV was transferred to a 2-ml plastic beaker covered with a lid, which contained 30 µl of TISAB III (Orion Research) prior to analysis. The samples were thoroughly mixed by vibration for 10 s and then analysed.

Statistical methods

The sample size chosen was based upon a simple power analysis that was performed before the start of the study and some earlier studies by Kashani et al, 1995 and Särner et al, 2003, where statistically significant differences were obtained with

Table 2 The results from Series I *in vitro*. The accumulated release of F for 60 min from fresh and old Miswaks impregnated in 0.01%, 0.1%, 0.5%, 1% and 3% NaF (mean ± SD of 10 samples/test)

NaF impregnation solution (%)	Release of F (ppm)				
	0 min	2 min	10 min	30 min	60 min
0.01%					
Fresh	0	0.09 ± 0.06	0.15 ± 0.05	0.35 ± 0.19	0.64 ± 0.41
Old	0	0.05 ± 0.01	0.17 ± 0.09	0.36 ± 0.23	0.54 ± 0.38
0.1%					
Fresh	0	0.79 ± 0.25	2.98 ± 1.49	8.96 ± 4.87	13.31 ± 4.63
Old	0	1.17 ± 0.49	3.23 ± 1.15	8.41 ± 2.70	11.72 ± 3.32
0.5%					
Fresh	0	1.35 ± 0.63	4.57 ± 1.77	10.25 ± 1.92	15.58 ± 3.87
Old	0	1.91 ± 0.85	4.24 ± 1.12	9.04 ± 2.79	14.40 ± 2.70
1%					
Fresh	0	2.00 ± 0.78	5.95 ± 1.93	12.66 ± 3.51	25.94 ± 13.74
Old	0	2.25 ± 1.74	7.41 ± 11.36	15.73 ± 12.57	19.22 ± 18.18
3%					
Fresh	0	7.13 ± 5.33	20.52 ± 14.15	41.18 ± 26.73	56.54 ± 35.80
Old	0	5.26 ± 3.88	14.85 ± 13.51	35.35 ± 33.82	46.09 ± 39.58

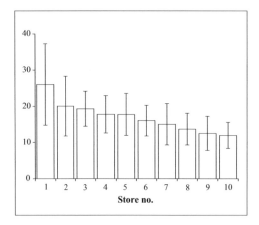

Fig 2 The F release *in vitro*, given in ranking order, from Miswaks purchased at 10 different stores (Series II). They were fluoridated in 0.5% NaF for 1 day. Only the 60-min F values are shown (mean ± SD of 10 pieces/test).

six individuals. Because of this, it was decided to include 10 subjects in the present study. An unpaired *t* test was applied on the 60-min *F* values *in vitro* to compare the old and the fresh Miswaks, as well as the Miswaks that were purchased from different stores. For Series II and IV *in vivo*, Kaleida-Graph version 4.0 was used to calculate the area under the curve (AUC) for each individual and each treatment. Statistical comparisons were made using two-way analysis of variance (ANOVA), followed by a multiple comparison test with Fisher's PLSD. For Series I and III *in vivo*, two-way ANOVA was also carried out on the F retention values. A value of $P < 0.05$ was considered to be statistically significant.

RESULTS

In vitro studies

The mean ± SD of the F release in Series I are shown in Table 2. There were large standard deviations (SDs). The results show that the higher the concentration of NaF in the impregnation solution, the more F was released from the Miswak, with a clear dose-response effect. There was no detectable F in the Miswaks at 0 min. The release of F was rapid, especially during the first 10 min. Fresh Miswaks showed a slightly higher F release than old Miswaks, especially at high NaF concentrations (i.e. at 1% and 3% NaF). However, there were no statistically significant differences between fresh and old Miswaks at 60 min for any of the five NaF concentrations.

The result from Series II is presented as means ± SD in Figure 2; only the 60-min values are shown. There were statistically significant differences between store 1 on one hand and stores 8, 9 and 10 on the other hand ($P < 0.05$).

Table 3 The results from Series I and Series III *in vivo*. Both the total volume of saliva (ml), collected during the 12-min period, and the F concentration (ppm) in saliva using a mouthrinse with 20 ml of water are shown. The 'F retention' was calculated as ml saliva × ppm F and expressed as mg F (mean ± SD and range of 10 individuals)

NaF impregnation solution (%)	Saliva + water rinse		'Fluoride retention' (mg F)*	
	Volume (ml)	F (ppm)	Mean ± SD	Range
0.01	27.6 ± 4.6	0.3 ± 0.1	0.01 ± 0.01	0.00–0.03
0.1	27.7 ± 4.8	7.7 ± 3.6	0.21 ± 0.11	0.06–0.44
0.3	29.0 ± 5.5	10.6 ± 2.7	0.31 ± 0.09	0.22–0.46
0.5	28.1 ± 5.7	14.0 ± 5.6	0.39 ± 0.13	0.21–0.61
1	29.0 ± 5.0	16.6 ± 9.9	0.48 ± 0.25	0.16–0.78
3	29.1 ± 5.0	31.1 ± 17.1	0.91 ± 0.50	0.22–1.80

*Calculated as volume (ml) × ppm F/1000 = mg F.

In vivo studies

The data in Table 3 show the mean ± SD for the oral F retention, which is expressed as milligram F for 6 of the 11 different NaF impregnation solutions. About 27 to 29 ml saliva was collected during the 12-min period, including the final mouthrinse with 20 ml of water. The calculated F retention increased at higher NaF impregnation concentrations. At 0.1% NaF, the mean was 0.21 mg F (range 0.06 to 0.44), and at 0.5% NaF it was about twice as much, that is, 0.39 mg F (range 0.21 to 0.61).

The data in Figure 3 show the mean salivary F concentration and the AUC values for both Series II and IV. Miswaks fluoridated in 0.1% to 0.3% NaF gave about the same F level as brushing with an F-containing dentifrice. The mean AUC in Series II was twice as high for the Miswak fluoridated in 3% NaF compared with that in 0.5% NaF ($P < 0.0001$) and four times higher compared with that in 0.1% NaF ($P < 0.0001$). In Series IV, the mean AUC was three times as high for Miswak impregnated in 0.5% NaF compared with that in 0.05% NaF and twice as high compared with that in 0.1% NaF. None of these differences in Series IV were, however, statistically significant (because of large SDs).

DISCUSSION

The present study shows that the release of F from NaF-impregnated Miswaks is a fast process both *in vitro* and *in vivo*. The quick release may be explained by the fact that the porous wood in *S. persica* can absorb and retain the NaF solution both on the surface (bark) and in porosities of the inner spongy part (pulp) (Baeshen et al, 2008). The retention and release of F depend on several factors, such as the degree of porosity and the nature of a Miswak. Morphological studies of Miswaks show that the plants are indeed very spongy (Al-Otaibi, 2004). All of these factors may influence the retention of NaF crystals that easily dissolve when coming into contact with a liquid, such as saliva and water. It is, therefore, an advantage to moisten the fluoridated Miswaks in the mouth for a few seconds just before they are used to speed up the F release process.

In vitro, there was a clear dose-response effect with respect to F release in water and NaF concentration of the impregnation solutions. Thus, the higher the concentration of NaF, the more F was released from the Miswak. These results are in agreement with those of the studies on fluoridated wooden toothpicks that were carried out in the authors' laboratory (Kashani et al, 1995) and on fluoridated Miswaks (Baeshen et al, 2008). There was also a slightly higher release of F from the fresh than from the old Miswaks, even if no statistically significant difference was observed. Both types are sold on the open market, but the fresh Miswaks are better tasting and somewhat more expensive. Moreover, there were large differences in F release between the Miswaks purchased from different stores, with a factor of approximately 2. The reason for this variation could be that some of the stores mostly sell fresh Miswaks, whereas others sell older types. The difference may also depend on the properties of the Miswak itself, as pointed out above, even if an attempt was made to control for both size and weight of the pieces in the present study.

When using a fluoridated Miswak, a relatively large surface area of the chewing stick will come into

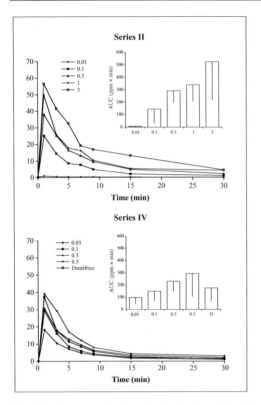

Fig 3 The F concentration in saliva *in vivo* from Series II (0.01%, 0.1%, 0.5%, 1% and 3% NaF) and Series IV (0.05%, 0.1%, 0.3%, 0.5% and dentifrice; the data from 0.2% and 0.4% are not shown). The bars show the AUC values (mean and SD only in one direction; *n* = 10).

contact with saliva. This means that F is released into the oral cavity and then subsequently swallowed. In the *in vivo* experiments (Series I and III), Miswaks fluoridated with 0.5% NaF for a day gave a mean F retention of 0.39 mg. As Miswak is used up to five times a day, around 2 mg of F will be swallowed every day. This amount can be considered safe from a toxicological point of view. However, to be on the safe side, and because of the great individual range, fluoridation in 0.1% NaF could be recommended resulting in an intake of $0.21 \times 5 \approx 1$ mg of F, as shown in Table 3. When comparing the F concentration in saliva expressed as AUC, about twice more F in saliva was found for Miswaks impregnated in 0.5% NaF compared with that in 0.32% NaF-containing dentifrice. For 0.1% NaF, the values were about the same as that for an F-containing dentifrice.

It has to be remembered that all of the F from the Miswak will be swallowed in contrast to F from the dentifrice.

Miswaks are commonly used in many Arab countries, such as Saudi Arabia, which have a high prevalence of dental caries (Al Dosari et al, 2004). Therefore, the authors believe that NaF-impregnated Miswaks may be a useful tool for the prevention of caries in these countries. This is of special interest from a cariological point of view, because Miswaks are used prior to each prayer, which means up to five times every day. Some individuals even use the Miswaks after eating, which may be favourable for the prevention of dental caries. It should also be pointed out that every time a Miswak is used, the old part is cut off and a new fresh part is peeled off and ready for brushing, which is favourable for F release.

In conclusion, NaF-impregnated Miswaks showed a quick release of F *in vitro* as well as *in vivo*. The authors therefore found that this type of chewing stick is an interesting F vehicle in those countries where they are commonly used. If they will be used in the future on a broad scale, it is recommended to use fresh Miswaks impregnated in 0.1% NaF or a maximum of 0.5% NaF for a day. Further clinical studies on fluoridated Miswaks should be carried out, however, for evaluating their caries-preventive effect.

ACKNOWLEDGEMENT

The authors would like to thank Ann-Britt Lundberg for her technical assistance. This study was part of a project supported by scholarship from the Saudi Arabian Ministry of Higher Education.

REFERENCES

1. Al Dosari AM, Wyne AH, Akpata ES, Khan NB. Caries prevalence and its relation to water fluoride levels among schoolchildren in central province of Saudi Arabia. Int Dent J 2004;54:424–428.

2. Almas K. The antimicrobial effects of seven different types of Asian chewing sticks. Trop Dent J 2001;24:17–20.

3. Almas K, Al-Zeid Z. The immediate antimicrobial effect of a toothbrush and Miswak on cariogenic bacteria: a clinical study. J Contemp Dent Pract 2004;5:105–114.

4. Almas K, Albaker A, Felemban N. Knowledge of dental health and diseases among dental patients, a multicenter study in Saudi Arabia. Indian J Dent Res 2000;11:145–155.

5. Al-Otaibi M. The Miswak (chewing stick) and oral health. Studies on oral hygiene practices of urban Saudi Arabia. Swed Dent J Suppl 2004;167:2–75.

6. Al-Otaibi M, Zimmerman M, Angmar-Månsson B. Prevailing oral hygiene practices among urban Saudi Arabians in relation to age, gender and socio-economic background. Acta Odontol Scand 2003;61:212–216.

7. Al-Otaibi M, Al-Harthy M, Gustafsson A, Johansson A, Claesson R, Angmar-Månsson B. Subgingival plaque microbiota in Saudi Arabians after use of Miswak chewing stick and toothbrush. J Clin Periodontol 2004;31:1048–1053.

8. Asadi SGR, Asadi ZG. Chewing sticks and the oral hygiene habits of adult Pakistani population. Int Dent J 1997;47:275–278.

9. Baeshen H, Kjellberg H, Lingström P, Birkhed D. Uptake and release of fluoride from fluoride impregnated chewing sticks (Miswaks) *in vitro* and *in vivo*. Caries Res 2008;42:363–368.

10. Boghani CP. Morbidity pattern of dental health problems. J Indian Dent Assoc 1978;50:277–281.

11. Darout IA, Albandar JM, Skaug N, Ali RW. Salivary microbiota levels in relation to periodontal status, experience of caries and Miswak use in Sudanese adults. J Clin Periodontol 2002;29:411–420.

12. Darout IA, Skuag N, Albandar JM. Subgingival microbiota levels and their associations with periodontal status at the sampled sites in an adult Sudanese population using Miswak or toothbrush regularly. Acta Odontol Scand 2003;61:115–122.

13. Elvin-Lewis M, Hall JB, Adu-Tuto M, Afful Y, Asante-Appiah K, Lieberman D. The dental health of chewing stick users of southern Ghana preliminary finding. J Prev Dent 1980;6:151–159.

14. Hardie J, Ahmed K. The Miswak as an aid in oral hygiene. J Philip Dent Assoc 1995;47:33–38.

15. Hattab FN. Miswak: the natural toothbrush. J Clin Dent 1997;8:125–129.

16. Kashani H, Birkhed D, Petersson LG. Uptake and release of fluoride from birch and lime toothpicks. Eur J Oral Sci 1995; 103:112–115.

17. Kashani H, Birkhed D, Petersson LG. Fluoride concentration in the approximal area after using toothpicks and other fluoride-containing products. Eur J Oral Sci 1998;106: 564–570.

18. Khoory T. The use of chewing sticks in preventive oral hygiene. Clin Prev Dent 1983;5:11–14.

19. Mörch T, Bjørvatn K. Laboratory study of fluoride impregnated toothpicks. Scand J Dent Res 1981;89:499–505.

20. Petersen PE, Mzee MO. Oral health profile of schoolchildren, mothers and school teachers in Zanzibar. Community Dent Health 1998;15:256–262.

21. Särner B, Lingström P, Birkhed D. Fluoride release from NaF- and AmF-impregnated toothpicks and dental flosses *in vitro* and *in vivo*. Caries Res 2003;61:289–296.

22. Särner B, Birkhed D, Huysmans MC, Ruben JL, Fidler V, Lingström P. Effect of fluoridated toothpicks and dental flosses on enamel and dentine and on plaque composition *in situ*. Caries Res 2005;39:52–59.

23. World Health Organization. Preventive Methods and Programmes for Oral Diseases. Technical Report Series 713. Geneva: World Health Organization, 1987.

24. Wu CD, Darout IA, Skaug N. Chewing sticks: timeless natural toothbrushes for oral cleansing. J Period Res 2001;36:275–284.

III

Acta Odontologica Scandinavica, 2010; Early Online, 1–8

informa
healthcare

ORIGINAL ARTICLE

Oral fluoride retention in orthodontic patients with and without fixed appliances after using different fluoridated home-care products

HOSAM BAESHEN[1,2], HEIDRUN KJELLBERG[1] & DOWEN BIRKHED[2]

[1]*Department of Orthodontics and* [2]*Department of Cariology, Institute of Odontology, The Sahlgrenska Academy at the University of Gothenburg, Gothenburg, Sweden*

Abstract
Objective. To evaluate oral fluoride (F) retention after using fluoridated toothpastes, rinsing solutions and chewing sticks (Miswaks) in orthodontic patients with and without orthodontic appliances. ***Material and methods.*** Nine orthodontic patients, with a mean age of 16 years, were included in a randomized, cross-over, experimental study. Six different home-care F products, two NaF toothpastes (0.32% and 1.1%), two NaF mouthwash solutions (0.05% and 0.2%) and two NaF-impregnated Miswaks chewing sticks (0.05% and 0.5%), were used both during the orthodontic treatment and 1 week after debonding. Unstimulated whole saliva and approximal saliva were collected from two interdental sites, before and up to 60 min after using each product for 2 min. The retention of F was calculated as the area under the 60-min F-clearance curve (AUC). ***Results.*** In general, the F concentrations at the various sites were higher before than after debonding. Moreover, the products with a high F content (toothpaste, mouthwash and Miswaks) resulted in higher F retention than the corresponding products with a lower F content. In whole saliva, the highest AUC values were found in patients using 0.2% NaF mouthwash, followed by 1.1% NaF toothpaste ($p < 0.05$). In approximal saliva, the retention values were highest after using 0.5% NaF-impregnated Miswaks in patients wearing orthodontic appliances ($p < 0.001$). ***Conclusions.*** The insertion of fixed orthodontic appliances appears to favor oral F retention for all the tested home-care F products. In addition, products with a high F content increase oral F retention.

Key Words: *Approximal area, fluoride retention, fluoride solution, fluoride toothpaste, Miswaks, orthodontic patients, saliva*

Introduction

The prevalence of dental caries has declined in the Western world in recent decades, probably because of the widespread use of fluoride (F) toothpaste [1–3]. Adolescents treated with fixed orthodontic appliances may be regarded as a risk group for caries due to increased plaque accumulation, food retention and shifts in the oral microflora [4–6]. The incidence of enamel demineralization (white spot lesions), adjacent to the brackets, has been estimated to be 15%–85% [7,8]. The retention sites in orthodontic patients, such as brackets, arch wires, ligatures and elastics, may be regarded as a negative factor from a cariological point of view with respect to plaque accumulation and food retention [6]. On the other hand, they may be a positive factor when it comes to the retention of F [9,10].

Toothpaste is the most commonly used home-care F product. Supplementary F, in forms such as solutions, tablets, chewing gums and gels, is often recommended to orthodontic patients [11–13]. Fluoridated products have varying abilities to elevate the concentration and distribution of F in the oral cavity. Rinsing solutions and toothpaste considerably increase the F concentration in saliva [14,15]. Rinsing with F leads to an elevated F concentration in dental plaque for up to 3 h at least [14]. In many Muslim countries, Miswaks (chewing sticks) are used for cleaning purposes several times per day. A recent study in the eastern province of Saudi Arabia revealed that the use of Miswaks is about twice as common as that of toothbrushes among schoolchildren [16]. We have recently developed a procedure to impregnate Miswaks with F [17,18]. The data are promising and show that the release of F from the chewing stick

Correspondence: Dowen Birkhed, Department of Cariology, Institute of Odontology, University of Gothenburg, Medicinaregatan 12, Box 450, SE-405 30 Gothenburg, Sweden. Tel: +46 31 786 32 01. Fax: +46 31 82 57 33. E-mail: birkhed@odontologi.gu.se

(Received 18 November 2009; accepted 18 December 2009)

ISSN 0001-6357 print/ISSN 1502-3850 online © 2010 Informa UK Ltd. (Informa Healthcare, Taylor & Francis AS)
DOI: 10.3109/00016350903571723

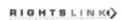

is a rapid process and thereby suitable for caries prevention.

Our hypothesis was that the oral F concentration, and thereby F retention, would be higher and more prolonged in patients with fixed orthodontic appliances than those without, for example when brushing the teeth with toothpaste or Miswaks or after using a rinsing solution. The aim was therefore to study the retention of F in the oral cavity, both in saliva and in the approximal area, after using different fluoridated home-care products, such as toothpastes, rinsing solutions and chewing sticks (Miswaks) in orthodontic patients with and without orthodontic appliances.

Material and methods

Subjects and study design

Nine orthodontic patients, two males and seven females, almost at the stage of debonding, were recruited from the specialist orthodontic clinics at the University of Gothenburg; their mean age was 16 years (range 14–19 years). They all had fixed orthodontic appliances in both the upper and lower jaws and had been treated due to bimaxillary crowding. The participants were scheduled for six visits with the appliances and another six shortly after debonding (i.e. without any appliances). The total study period for these 12 visits was 3 months (12 weeks). Figure 1 shows a schematic outline illustrating the design of the study. The Ethics Committee at the University of Gothenburg had approved the study (code number 355-09). Informed consent was obtained from the subjects before the start of the study.

F products

This experimental in situ study had a cross-over design, in which all nine participants used all six F products on two occasions in a randomized order. The washout period between each test was a minimum of 1 day. The participants were not allowed to use any fluoridated product on the day of examination. The following six products were included in the study: (1) toothpaste containing 0.32% NaF (Pepsodent; Lever Fabergé, Stockholm, Sweden); (2) toothpaste containing 1.1% NaF (Duraphat; Colgate Palmolive, Glostrup, Denmark); (3) mouthwash solution containing 0.05% NaF (Dentan; Meda, Stockholm, Sweden); (4) mouthwash solution containing 0.2% NaF (Dentan); (5) Miswaks impregnated in 0.05% NaF for 1 day at our laboratory; and (6) Miswaks impregnated for 1 day in 0.5% NaF. The impregnation procedure has recently been described in detail [17,18].

F administration

Before each test, the subjects chewed on paraffin wax for 5 min and rinsed with distilled water for 30 s.

Toothpaste. One g of paste was applied to a wet toothbrush and the subject brushed his/her teeth for 2 min. After brushing, the remaining toothpaste was spat out and the mouth was rinsed with 5 ml of water for 5 s.

Mouthwash solution. Ten ml of the solution was swirled around the mouth for 2 min with active movements of the cheeks and lips.

Miswaks. The cover was first removed and the participants then chewed on the stick for a short time (3–5 s), before it was moved around the dentition to clean all the buccal tooth surfaces and all the buccally oriented approximal surfaces, for 2 min, as described previously (Figures 2A and 2C) [17,18].

Sampling procedure

Resting whole saliva and approximal saliva from two sites were collected just before (0-min sample; baseline) and after 1, 3, 5, 10, 15, 30 and 60 min, making eight samples per test. In all, 2592 saliva samples were collected for the whole study (nine subjects×six

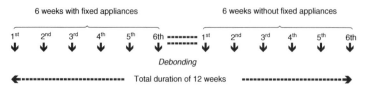

Once a week, nine patients tested six home-care F products in a randomized order: toothpaste 0.32% NaF, toothpaste 1.1% NaF, mouthwash solution 0.05% NaF, mouthwash solution 0.2% NaF, Miswaks impregnated for 1 day in 0.05% NaF and Miswaks impregnated for 1 day in 0.5% NaF

6 weeks with fixed appliances   6 weeks without fixed appliances

1ˢᵗ   2ⁿᵈ   3ʳᵈ   4ᵗʰ   5ᵗʰ   6ᵗʰ ------ 1ˢᵗ   2ⁿᵈ   3ʳᵈ   4ᵗʰ   5ᵗʰ   6ᵗʰ

Debonding

←·········· Total duration of 12 weeks ··········→

Figure 1. Schematic outline summarizing the design of the study.

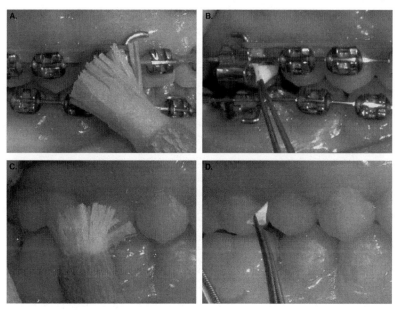

Figure 2. (A, C) Use of a Miswak for cleaning the teeth with and without orthodontic appliances. (B, D) Sampling of approximal saliva with triangular paper points is also shown.

products×three sites×eight time points×two occasions). Small, standardized, triangle-shaped paper points (base: 1.5 mm; length: 5 mm) were inserted in the two approximal areas (mesial 16 and mesial 25) for 30 s (Figure 2B and 2D) in order to suck up around 4 μl of saliva [19]. The paper points were then transferred to plastic Eppendorf tubes containing 200 μl of deionized water and 20 μl of Total Ionic Strength Adjuster Buffer (TISAB) III buffer solution (dilution 10:1; Thermo Electron, Waltham, MA, USA).

F analysis

Prior to the F analyses, the samples were mixed by vibration for 10 s. The F concentration was determined by means of an F-sensitive electrode connected to an expandable ion analyzer (Orion Research, Boston, MA, USA) by placing the surface of the electrode in close contact with the solution. Analysis of F concentration was performed using a set of standard solutions from 0.526 μM F (0.01 ppm) to 5.26 mM F (100 ppm), according to the manufacturer's instructions. The same technician analyzed all 2592 samples blindly.

Statistical analysis

A simplified power calculation was performed before starting the study. Means and standard deviations

(SDs) were calculated for each F product with and without the fixed orthodontic appliances. The area under the clearance curve for 0–60 min (AUC) was measured using the KaleidaGraph software program (Version 4.0; Synergy Software, Reading, PA, USA) for each individual and each product. The mean differences between the AUC values with and without orthodontic appliances and between the various products were compared using a paired *t*-test. $p < 0.05$ was considered to be statistically significant. Statistical comparisons using three-way ANOVA, followed by multiple comparison tests with Student–Newman–Keuls were also performed, which confirmed the result of the paired *t*-test.

Results

Generally, the F concentration values for all products and for all patients with fixed orthodontic appliances showed higher F retention than without the appliances.

Figure 3 shows the means and SDs of AUCs in saliva from the patients with orthodontic appliances; the six F products are given in ranking order. 0.2% NaF mouthwash and 1.1% NaF toothpaste produced the highest F values, which were significantly higher compared with the other four products ($p < 0.05$). The same ranking order was found without orthodontic appliances but with generally lower

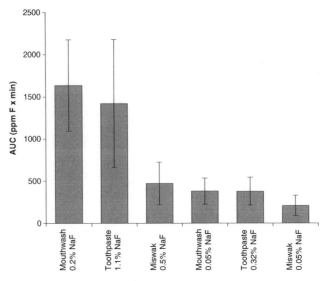

Figure 3. The AUC values (Mean ± SD) values of the F concentration in saliva from six different F products, arranged from the highest to the lowest F concentration, in patients ($n = 9$) wearing fixed orthodontic appliances.

F values compared with orthodontic appliances (data not shown).

Figure 4 shows the mean F concentrations during the 60 min and the AUC values in saliva and at the two approximal sites with orthodontic appliances. Only data for 0.2% NaF mouthwash solution, 1.1% NaF toothpaste and 0.5% NaF Miswaks are shown. The F concentration was high, especially during the first 10 min; there were no significant differences between the three sampling sites, except for Miswaks, which produced higher values at the two approximal sites than in whole saliva ($p < 0.05$). Both the F concentration and the AUC were about 1.5-times higher for 0.5% NaF-impregnated Miswaks compared with 0.2% NaF mouthwash solution and 0.5% NaF toothpaste ($p < 0.05$).

Figure 5 shows the AUC values for the two approximal sites with and without orthodontic appliances. Generally, in all the tests, the highest F release was obtained for mesial 25, followed by mesial 16 (even if the differences were not always statistically significant). Using 0.5% NaF-impregnated Miswaks, both with and without orthodontic appliances, resulted in the highest F retention in approximal saliva, especially at mesial 25, with statistically significant differences compared with all the other F products ($p < 0.001$).

Discussion

To our knowledge, there are no similar studies in the literature comparing oral F retention with and without

fixed appliances in orthodontic patients after using different home-care F products. The main result of the present investigation was that the F concentration for all products showed higher retention when patients wore the appliances. This held true both in whole saliva and at approximal sites. The three products tested in this study (toothpaste, mouthwash and Miswaks) were evaluated in forms with both a low and a high NaF concentration. As expected, the high-F products generally produced a higher salivary F concentration and higher AUC values than the low-F products on both test occasions, i.e. with and without orthodontic appliances. This may be an advantage from a cariological point of view, as oral F reservoirs on the teeth, oral mucosa and around the brackets can have a protective effect against caries [10].

The large variation in F retention between the products could be explained by the F concentrations in the products themselves, by the presence and absence of the orthodontic appliances and by the sampling site [20,21]. For example, 0.5% NaF Miswaks produced the highest values in the approximal area compared with all other products, followed by 0.2% NaF mouthwash solution. On the other hand, 0.2% NaF mouthwash solution and 1.1% NaF toothpaste produced the highest values in whole saliva.

The preventive effect of rinsing with F on dental caries has been reported in several studies [22–24]. The fact that the mouthwash solution raised F concentrations more than toothpaste or Miswaks indicates that the F distribution in the oral cavity was

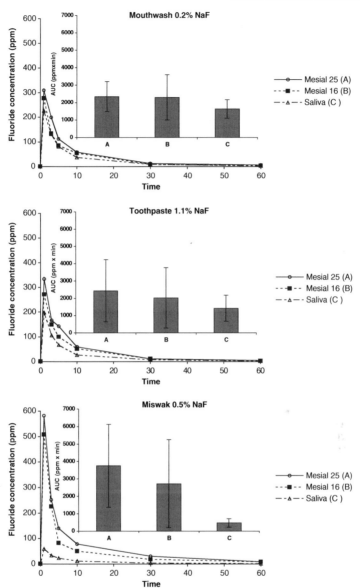

Figure 4. Mean values (*n* = 9) of F concentration both in saliva and at two approximal sites up to 60 min after using three F products (0.2% NaF mouthwash, 1.1% NaF toothpaste and 0.5% NaF-impregnated Miswaks) in orthodontic patients with fixed appliances. The AUC values (0–60 min), expressed as the mean ± SD are also inset.

more complete. This is in agreement with a recent study [25] which showed that rinsing with NaF resulted in higher approximal F concentrations compared with fluoridated toothpicks and dental flosses. The reason why the mouthwash is more powerful in terms of F retention than other products may be that it

penetrates different areas, such as between the brackets and wires, more easily when swirled around the mouth.

We have recently studied F uptake and release from NaF-impregnated Miswaks and found that the release is a rapid process [17,18]. The use of fluoridated

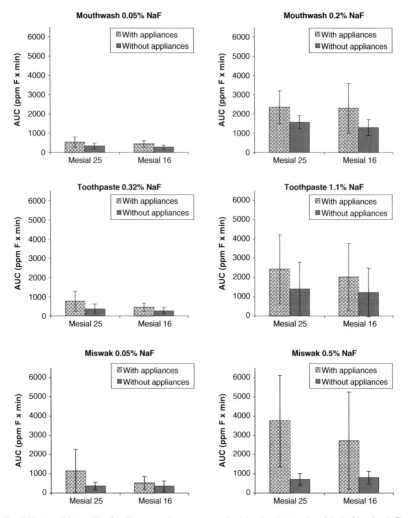

Figure 5. The AUC values (Mean ± SD) of the F concentration at two approximal sites (mesial 25 and mesial 16) after using six F products in orthodontic patients ($n = 9$) with and without fixed appliances.

Miswaks may not only be restricted to poor countries; it can also be applied in modern countries by patients with orthodontic appliances. The F-containing bristles appear to increase oral F retention, especially between the brackets. The present results showed that 0.5% NaF Miswaks produced F retention that was 1.5-times higher than 0.2% NaF mouthwash solution and 0.5% NaF toothpaste in approximal saliva. Another advantage of Miswaks is that there is no need for post-brushing water rinsing as there is after using toothpaste.

A systematic review by Twetman *et al.* [26] in 2003 reported strong scientific evidence showing that the daily use of F toothpaste is an effective method for preventing dental caries. Several studies indicate that there is a more or less linear relationship between the F concentration in the toothpastes and the extent of caries reduction [15,27,28]. Various factors, including the concentration of F in the paste, the amount of toothpaste applied to the brush, the frequency of brushing and post-brushing water rinsing, influence the efficacy of F toothpaste [29]. Adults and teenagers with a high risk of caries are suitable target groups for using a dentifrice containing 5000 ppm F (equal to 1.1% NaF). Adolescents run an increased risk of caries when their teeth have just erupted. A dentifrice with a high F content, like the one used in the present study, has also been recommended for optimal caries prevention strategies during orthodontic treatment [12]. An interesting observation made recently is that post-brushing water rinsing has a negative impact on the retention of F in the approximal area [15]. This can be extended to orthodontic patients, who should be advised to use just a minimum amount of water after brushing their teeth with F toothpaste.

It seems logical that the residual volume of saliva and salivary flow increase after insertion of fixed orthodontic appliances [30] and that those two factors may shorten the F retention time in the oral cavity. The appliance consists of many retentive components that provide numerous recesses where F may be trapped. The present study showed that F retention was somewhat prolonged for patients with than without appliances. It should be remembered that in most cases these differences were rather small.

In conclusion, the retention of F from fluoridated mouthwash solution, toothpaste and Miswaks is somewhat more pronounced in patients with orthodontic appliances than without. Products with a high F concentration may have a favorable effect on orthodontic patients as they considerably increase the retention of F. Moreover, fluoridated Miswaks is an interesting product in orthodontic patients in countries where it is used frequently, since it has a 'dual effect', i.e. both brushing and F delivery.

Acknowledgements

The authors thank Professor Emerita Birgit Thilander for valuable discussions, Ms. Ann-Britt Lundberg for technical assistance and Dr. Tommy Johansson for statistical assistance.

This study was a part of a project supported by a scholarship from the Saudi Arabian Ministry of Higher Education.

Declaration of interest: The authors report no conflicts of interest. The authors alone are responsible for the content and writing of the paper.

References

[1] Bratthall D, Hänsel-Petersson G, Sundberg H. Reasons for the caries decline: what do the experts believe? Eur J Oral Sci 1996;104:416–22.

[2] WHO. WHO oral health report. Continuous improvement of oral health in the 21st century. The approach of the WHO Global Oral Health Programme. Geneva, Switzerland: World Health Organization; 2003.

[3] Marinho VC, Higgins JP, Sheiham A, Logans S. Fluoride toothpastes for preventing dental caries in children and adolescents. Cochrane Database Syst Rev 2003;1:CD002278.

[4] Sandham HJ, Nadeau L, Phillips HI. The effect of chlorhexidine varnish treatment on salivary mutans streptococcal levels in child orthodontic patients. J Dent Res 1992;71:32–5.

[5] Chang HS, Walsh LJ, Freer TJ. The effect of orthodontic treatment on salivary flow, pH, buffer capacity, and levels of mutans streptococci and lactobacilli. Aust Orthod J 1999; 15:229–34.

[6] Türkkahraman H, Sayin MO, Bozkurt FY, Yetkin Z, Kaya S, Onal S. Archwire ligation techniques, microbial colonization, and periodontal status in orthodontically treated patients. Angle Orthod 2005;75:231–6.

[7] Mitchell L. Decalcification during orthodontic treatment with fixed appliances—an overview. Br J Orthod 1992;19: 199–205.

[8] Fornell AC, Sköld-Larsson K, Hallgren A, Bergstrand F, Twetman S. Effect of a hydrophobic tooth coating on gingival health, mutans streptococci, and enamel demineralization in adolescents with fixed orthodontic appliances. Acta Odontol Scand 2002;60:37–41.

[9] Ekstrand J, Lagerlöf F, Oliveby A. Some aspects of the kinetics of fluoride in saliva. In: Leach SA, editor. Factors relating to demineralisation and remineralisation of the teeth. Oxford, UK: IRL Press; 1986. p. 91–8.

[10] Duckworth RM, Morgan SN, Ingram GS, Page DJ. Oral fluoride reservoirs and their relationship to anticaries efficacy. In: Embery G, Rølla G, editors. Clinical and biological aspects of dentifrices. New York: Oxford University Press; 1992. p. 91–104.

[11] Benson PE, Shah AA, Millett DT, Dyer F, Parkin N, Vine RS. Fluorides, orthodontics and demineralization: a systematic review. J Orthod 2005;32:102–14.

[12] Derks A, Katsaros C, Frencken JE, van't Hof MA, Kuijpers-Jagtman AM. Caries-inhibiting effect of preventive measures during orthodontic treatment with fixed appliances. A systematic review. Caries Res 2004;38:413–20.

[13] Benson PE, Parkin N, Millett DT, Dyer FE, Vine S, Shah A. Fluorides for the prevention of white spots on teeth during fixed brace treatment. Cochrane Database Syst Rev 2004;3: CD003809.

[14] Seppä L, Salmenkivi S, Hausen H. Salivary fluoride concentration in adults after different fluoride procedures. Acta Odontol Scand 1997;55:84–7.

[15] Nordström A, Birkhed D. Fluoride retention in approximal plaque and saliva using two NaF dentifrices containing 5,000 and 1,450 ppm F with and without water rinsing. Caries Res 2009;43:64–9.

[16] Amin TT, Al-Abad BM. Oral hygiene practices, dental knowledge, dietary habits and their relation to caries among male primary school children in Al Hassa, Saudi Arabia. Int J Dent Hyg 2008;6:361–70.

[17] Baeshen H, Kjellberg H, Lingström P, Birkhed D. Uptake and release of fluoride from fluoride impregnated chewing sticks (Miswaks) in vitro and in vivo. Caries Res 2008;42: 363–8.

[18] Baeshen H, Birkhed D. Release of fluoride from fresh and old NaF-impregnated chewing sticks (Miswaks) in vitro and oral retention in vivo. Oral Health Prev Dent 2010; In press.

[19] Kashani H, Birkhed D, Petersson LG. Fluoride concentration in the approximal area after using toothpicks and other fluoride-containing products. Eur J Oral Sci 1998;106: 564–70.

[20] Gabre P, Birkhed D, Gahnberg L. Fluoride retention of a mucosa adhesive paste compared with other home-care fluoride products. Caries Res 2008;42:240–6.

[21] Sjögren K, Birkhed D. Effect of various postbrushing activities on salivary fluoride concentration after tooth brushing with a sodium fluoride dentifrice. Caries Res 1994;28:127–31.

[22] Marinho VC, Higgins JP, Logan S, Sheiham A. Fluoride mouthrinses for preventing dental caries in children and adolescents. Cochrane Database Syst Rev 2003;3: CD002284.

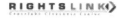

[23] Marinho VC, Higgins JP, Sheiham A, Logan S. One topical fluoride (toothpastes, or mouthrinses, or gels, or varnishes) versus another for preventing dental caries in children and adolescents. Cochrane Database Syst Rev 2004;1:CD002780.

[24] Fure S, Gahnberg L, Birkhed D. A comparison of four home-care fluoride programs on the caries incidence in the elderly. Gerodontology 1998;15:51–60.

[25] Särner B, Lingström P, Birkhed D. Fluoride release from NaF- and AmF-impregnated toothpicks and dental flosses in vitro and in vivo. Acta Odontol Scand 2003;61:289–96.

[26] Twetman S, Axelsson S, Dahlgren H, Holm AK, Källestål C, Lagerlöf F, et al. Caries-preventive effect of fluoride toothpaste: a systematic review. Acta Odontol Scand 2003;61:347–55.

[27] Birkeland JM. Fluoride content of dental plaque after brushing with a fluoride dentifrice. Scand J Dent Res 1972;80:80–1.

[28] White DJ, Nancollas GH. Physical and chemical considerations of the role of firmly and loosely bound fluoride in caries prevention. J Dent Res 1990;69:634–6.

[29] Davies RM, Ellwood RP, Davies GM. The rational use of fluoride toothpaste. Int J Dent Hyg 2003;1:3–8.

[30] Forsberg CM, Oliveby A, Lagerlöf F. Salivary clearance of sugar before and after insertion of fixed orthodontic appliances. Am J Orthod Dentofac Orthop 1992;102:527–30.

IV

ORIGINAL ARTICLE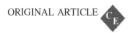

Effect of Fluoridated Miswaks (Chewing Sticks) on White Spot Lesions in Post-Orthodontic Patients Evaluated by the DIAGNOdent pen and ICDAS II

Hosam A. Baeshen[a], Peter Lingström[b], Dowen Birkhed[c]
Göteborg, Sweden

Introduction: This article illustrates a new treatment method and evaluates the effect of the frequent use of fluoridated Miswaks on the remineralization of white spot lesions (WSL), diagnosed at debonding. **Methods:** Thirty-seven orthodontic patients (mean age 17.2 years), with a minimum of 4 WSL on the buccal surfaces of the upper incisors, canines, premolars and first molars after completing orthodontic therapy, were enrolled in a double-blind, randomized, longitudinal trial lasting 6 weeks. The subjects were divided into two groups using: a) fluoridated Miswaks impregnated in 0.5% NaF (test group, n=19) and b) non-fluoridated Miswaks (control group, n=18). A custom-made mouth tray, covering half the dentition in the upper jaw, was used while brushing with the Miswaks 5 times/day. The WSL were scored using a DIAGNOdent pen, as well as the International Caries Detection and Assessment System (ICDAS II) index, at baseline and 2, 4 and 6 weeks after debonding. **Results:** Both the DIAGNOdent readings and the ICDAS II index of the WSL decreased in the test group on the uncovered side of the dentition but not on the covered side during the 6-week trial ($P <0.0001$). There was also a slight improvement in the control group (ns). There was a strong correlation between the DIAGNOdent values and the ICDAS II index when all the data were pooled ($P <0.01$). **Conclusions:** The frequent use of fluoridated Miswaks had a remineralizing effect on WSL. The DIAGNOdent pen may be a useful tool for diagnosing and monitoring WSL over a relatively short period of time. (Am J Orthod Dentofacial Orthop 2010;00:00)

Caries lesions on smooth surfaces are commonly found among patients with

[a] Orthodontist and PhD resident, Departments of Cariology and Orthodontics, Institute of Odontology, The Sahlgrenska Academy, University of Gothenburg, Göteborg, Sweden
[b] Professor, Department of Cariology, Institute of Odontology, The Sahlgrenska Academy, University of Gothenburg, Göteborg, Sweden
[c] Professor and Chairman, Department of Cariology, Institute of Odontology, The Sahlgrenska Academy, University of Gothenburg, Göteborg, Sweden

Corresponding author: Professor Dowen Birkhed, Department of Cariology, Institute of Odontology, The Sahlgrenska Academy, University of Gothenburg, Box 450, SE-405 30 Göteborg, Sweden
(e-mail: birkhed@odontologi.gu.se)

high caries activity during and after orthodontic treatment.[1,2] Studies have shown that white spot lesions (WSL) can develop as quickly as within one month after bonding.[3,4] The prevalence of WSL after orthodontic treatment varies in different studies.[1,2,5,6] Minor lesions may be esthetically disturbing and often remain after the treatment[7,8], while advanced lesions may even require restorative treatment.[1,9] This problem can be minimized by preventive treatment using fluoride (F) toothpaste and rinsing solutions, oral hygiene instructions and topical F application.

The clinical diagnosis of WSL has been made primarily using traditional methods, such as visual inspection after air drying and tactile examination by dental probing. However, the subjectivity, lack of reproducibility and prerequisite of the presence of a significantly advanced lesion have led to the introduction of several optical devices in recent decades. One such technique is laser fluorescence.[10] The results of recent studies suggest that this technique may be appropriate for the early detection and assessment of WSL in orthodontic patients.[11,12]

A new clinical index, the International Caries Detection and Assessment System (ICDAS), was developed with the aim of designing an internationally accepted caries detection system that would also enable the assessment of early enamel demineralization.[13] In the ICDAS I (2003), the visual examination was carried out on clean, plaque-free teeth after careful drying. The criteria were subsequently modified and the ICDAS II was created. The improvement consisted of an exchange of codes to ensure that the system would reflect increased severity.[13,14]

Miswaks (chewing sticks) are used in many countries around the world for cleaning purposes and are often used up to 5 times/day. We have recently developed a procedure to impregnate Miswaks with F.[15,16] The data reveal that the F release from the chewing stick is a rapid process and the Miswaks are thereby suitable for caries prevention. The advantage of fluoridated Miswaks is that they have a "dual effect", i.e. firstly cleaning the buccal surfaces and secondly producing a high F concentration around the teeth. The aims of the present study were: 1) to evaluate the effect of the frequent use of fluoridated Miswaks on the remineralization of WSL diagnosed at debonding and 2) to compare the two diagnostic methods, laser fluorescence and the ICDAS II.

MATERIALS AND METHODS

Experimental design

Thirty-seven orthodontic patients, 11 males and 26 females, with a mean age of 17.2 years, were recruited from three different dental hospitals in Jeddah, Saudi Arabia: 1) the King Fahad Armed Forces Hospital, 2) the King Faisal Specialist Hospital and Research Center and 3) the King Fahad General Hospital. Figure 1 shows the schematic design of the study. The subjects were selected from a group of orthodontic patients who had full fixed appliance therapy (straight wire appliances) due to bimaxillary crowding, with a mean treatment period of 18 months. The inclusion criterion was at least 2 WSL on both the left and right side of the dentition in the upper jaw (16-26), adjacent to the site of the orthodontic band or bracket, i.e. a minimum of 4 WSL/subject (total of 152 WSL in the test group and 140 WSL in the control group). Ethical approval was obtained before starting the study.

All the participants and their parents were informed about the study and written consent was obtained before the start. After debonding and debanding, and at each visit, full-mouth cleaning with a rotating rubber cup, using pumice and water, and, if necessary, professional supragingival scaling, was performed to remove plaque, calculus and any remaining composite bonding material. Care was taken to avoid disturbing the WSL that were going to be evaluated.

The study was performed as a double-blind, longitudinal trial lasting 6 weeks. The participants were randomly divided into two groups: 1) a test group with 19 patients using fluoridated Miswaks impregnated in 0.5% NaF and 2) a control group with 18 patients using non-fluoridated Miswaks.

The Miswaks were impregnated in 0.5% NaF as previously described in detail by Baeshen et al. (2008).[15] The two types of Miswak were identical apart from their F content. They were packed in plastic bags and coded.

The chewing sticks for both groups were used on one side of the upper jaw, 5 times a day for 6 weeks; special attention was paid to the WSL. An individual plastic mouth tray (Essix, Dentsply, Parkland, USA) covering half the dentition was used, as shown in Figure 2. The tray was applied to the teeth immediately after toothbrushing and was kept in place while using the Miswak and for a minimum of 30 minutes afterwards. Written instructions, with photo illustrations, were also given to the patient and his/her parent to ensure that the Miswak and the mouth tray were used correctly. All the subjects were told to use fluoridated toothpaste (1450 ppm F, Signal 2, Binzagr Unilever, Jeddah, Saudi Arabia) twice a day, but they were instructed to use no other F products during the 6-week trial.

White spot lesions (WSL)

At baseline (debonding visit) and 2, 4 and 6 weeks after debonding, the WSL were scored using two different methods: 1) DIAGNOdent pen (KaVo, Biberach, Germany) and 2) visual examination using the ICDAS II index. The buccal surfaces of all the test teeth were photographed with a digital camera (Fujifilm FinePix S3 Pro SLR; Fuji Photo Film, Tokyo, Japan), equipped with a 105-mm macro lens and a ring flash with cross-polarization filters. The intra-oral photos (one front and one for each side) were taken on each visit (Fig 3). The same examiner (H.B.) performed all the measurements.

DIAGNOdent pen measurements

The same DIAGNOdent pen device was used throughout the study. Before each session, the instrument was calibrated against the ceramic standard, supplied by the manufacturer, and then calibrated for each individual by measuring a sound area of the buccal surface.[10,11] The surface was dried with compressed air for 5 seconds prior to measurement, which was made for 10 seconds. Each buccal surface was divided into three areas: 1) mesial, 2) center and 3) distal. Each site was scanned three times by the pen, using probe tip 2, and the highest value from the three readings was registered.

Visual examination (ICDAS II index)

Visual examination was performed immediately at debonding. The buccal surfaces of the test teeth were examined and recorded on each visit using the ICDAS II index. This was done after drying the tooth surfaces for 5 seconds with compressed air. The assessment was performed with the aid of a mouth mirror and a blunt probe under clinical lighting, according to ICDAS II index criteria, presented in Table I.

Blinding

The participants and the examiner were not aware of the group assignment, not even the covered or non-covered side, to ensure the complete double-blindness of the study. No records of the readings from the previous registrations were available at any of the follow-up measurements.

Data analysis and statistics

A power analysis was performed before the start of the study with an assumption significance level of 0.01, standard deviation of 3.0, least detectable difference of 4.0 (based on DIAGNOdent pen values) and a power for that detection of 90%. A sample size of 17 patients/group was suggested. The "within factors" were time (four time points) and quadrant (covered and non-covered), while the "between factor" was treatment group (fluoridated and non-fluoridated Miswaks).

Means and standard deviations were calculated for each visit and patient for both ICDAS and DIAGNOdent pen measurements. The mean values were calculated for the teeth in one and the same quadrant. The mean changes (Δ) at baseline and at 6 weeks for the covered and non-covered sides were analyzed using a paired t-test. For comparisons between the test and control group, a non-paired t-test was used. As a multiple t-test was used, a statistically significant difference of P <0.01 was accepted. The correlation between the ICDAS II index score and the DIAGNOdent readings at baseline and at 6 weeks was analyzed using Pearson's correlation coefficient.

Twenty percent of the measurements for both the ICDAS II scores and DIAGNOdent readings were recorded twice by the same examiner (H.B.). Cross-tabulation revealed that 91% of the ICDAS II readings were the same, while 9% revealed a difference of ±1 score only. When it came to the DIAGNOdent readings, 84% were the same, with ±1 readings for 14.5% and ±2 readings for 1.5%.

RESULTS

During the 6-week trial, a total of 404 teeth were examined. Table II shows the DIAGNOdent pen and ICDAS II index values at baseline and 6 weeks and the differences between the two visits. There were statistically significant differences between the two quadrants in the test group (P <0.0001) but not in the control group.

Figures 4 and 5 show the means and standard deviations of the readings from the DIAGNOdent pen and ICDAS II index at baseline and after 2, 4 and 6 weeks, for both covered and non-covered quadrants. There was a gradual decrease for non-covered surfaces treated with fluoridated Miswaks. There was also a minor decrease for the covered surfaces in the test group. In the control group, the values for the two sides stayed more or less the same.

Pearson's correlation coefficient between the ICDAS II index scores and the DIAGNOdent pen readings at 6 weeks was

0.76 (P <0.001), as shown in Figure 6. A similar correlation was found at baseline and at 2 and 4 weeks (data not shown).

DISCUSSION

In the present study, WSL that formed around fixed appliances during orthodontic treatment were followed longitudinally over a period of 6 weeks. During this experimental period, both the DIAGNOdent pen readings and the clinical index values decreased in the test group, indicating the remineralization of the caries lesions. This effect is probably mostly related to the release of F from the Miswaks, since the remineralization effect was much smaller in the control group using non-fluoridated Miswaks. Another interesting finding was that the DIAGNOdent pen was found to be a useful and reproducible method that could be used to quantify WSL and to test the effectiveness of a preventive regimen.

We have recently studied the F uptake and release from NaF-impregnated Miswaks and found that the release is a rapid process.[15,16] The use of fluoridated Miswaks may not only be restricted to certain countries but can also be applied in all countries by patients with orthodontic appliances.[17] The F-containing bristles easily reach the buccal surfaces of the teeth. Another advantage of using fluoridated Miswaks is that there is no need for post-brushing water rinsing, as there is after using F toothpaste, which has been found to have a negative impact on oral F retention.[18]

The slight decrease in the WSL that was also seen in the covered sites in the test subjects using the fluoridated Miswaks indicates that the mouth tray did not totally prevent F reaching the buccal surfaces on the contralateral side of the dentition. However, even when this is taken into account, the effect was still much greater at the treated sites.

The ICDAS II index was included in the present investigation in order to be compared with the DIAGNOdent pen. It was found that the clinical index correlated well with the DIAGNOdent values (r=0.76). So the progression/regression of WSL can be registered using both methods, even during such a short period as 6 weeks. We therefore believe that both the ICDAS II and the DIAGNOdent pen are useful for longitudinal studies *in vivo*. However, the advantage of the pen is that the readings can be shown to the patient and may therefore have a pedagogic value. The advantages of using the ICDAS II is that it is easy to use, inexpensive and less time consuming, but more subjective and less informative for the patient.[19] On the other hand, the DIAGNOdent pen is more informative for the patient and it is also easy to use and carry in the clinic, as well as being more accurate and reproducible[11,20], but the disadvantages are that it has a higher cost and is more time consuming.

Several studies have assessed the presence of WSL using photographic techniques.[21,22] However, there is difficulty achieving consistency in lighting, reflection and angulation. In the present study, we attempted to standardize the light by using a ring flash with cross-polarization filters and by fixing the focal length distance of the lens at 50 cm. In spite of this, it was not possible to standardize the photos in order to score the WSL in an optimal manner, as shown in Figure 3.

The experimental period of 6 weeks used in the present investigation might be regarded as short compared with other studies.[7,23,24] For ethical reasons, all the participants were provided with F toothpaste for use twice daily. For this reason, the observed remineralization is a combination of factors. Since the control group was also given F toothpaste and used non-fluoridated Miswaks, we believe that the remineralization of WSL can be mainly attributed to the F release from the Miswaks.

CONCLUSIONS

1. Fluoridated Miswaks impregnated with 0.5% NaF have a remineralization effect on the WSL compared with non-fluoridated Miswaks.
2. Over a period of 6 weeks, it was possible to use both the DIAGNOdent pen and a clinical caries index (ICDAS II) to quantify the remineralization of WSL.

The authors would like to extend their thanks to Major General Mohammed Al Halafi, Dr. Yasser Rhbeini and Dr. Majed Alborney from the King Fahad Armed Forces Hospital, Dr. Tarek Al-Jehani and Dr. Mohammed Yasser Al-Tabbaa from the King Faisal Specialist Hospital and Research Center and Dr. Fawzi Al-Ghamdi, Dr. Jamal Al-Gahtani, Dr. Hakeem Mushtaq and Dr. Reem Qalei from the King Fahad General Hospital. Special thanks to Tommy Johansson for his statistical assistance.
This Study was a part of a project supported by a scholarship from the Saudi Arabian Ministry of Higher Education.

REFERENCES

1. Gorton J, Featherstone JD. In vivo inhibition of demineralization around orthodontic brackets. Am J Orthod Dentofacial Orthop 2003;123:10-14.
2. Boersma JG, Van der Veen MH, Lagerweij MD, Bokhout B, Prahl-Andersen B. Caries prevalence measured with QLF after treatment with fixed orthodontic appliances: influencing factors. Caries Res 2005;39:41-47.
3. Øgaard B, Rölla G, Arends J. Orthodontic appliances and enamel demineralization. Part 1. Lesion development. Am J Orthod Dentofacial Orthop 1988;94:68-73.
4. Melrose CA, Appleton J, Lovius BB. A scanning electron microscopic study of early enamel caries formed in vivo beneath orthodontic bands. Br J Orthod 1996;23:43-47.
5. Gorelick L, Geiger AM, Gwinnett AJ. Incidence of white spot formation after bonding and banding. Am J Orthod Dentofacial Orthop 1982;81:93-98.
6. Øgaard B, Rölla G, Arends J, ten Cate JM. Orthodontic appliances and enamel demineralization. Part 2. Prevention and treatment of lesions. Am J Orthod Dentofacial Orthop 1988;94:123-128.
7. O'Reilly MM, Featherstone JD. Demineralization and remineralization around orthodontic appliances: an in vivo study. Am J Orthod Dentofacial Orthop 1987;92:33-40.
8. Årtun J, Brobakken BO. Prevalence of carious white spots after orthodontic treatment with multibonded appliances. Eur J Orthod 1986;8:229-234.
9. Basdra EK, Huber H, Komposch G. Fluoride released from orthodontic bonding agents alters the enamel surface and inhibits enamel demineralization in vitro. Am J Orthod Dentofacial Orthop 1996;109:466-472.
10. Lussi A, Imwinkelried S, Pitts N, Longbottom C, Reich E. Performance and reproducibility of a laser fluorescence system for detection of occlusal caries in vitro. Caries Res 1999;33:261-266.
11. Aljehani A, Yousif MA, Angmar-Månsson B, Shi XQ. Longitudinal quantification of incipient carious lesions in postorthodontic patients using a fluorescence method. Eur J Oral Sci 2006;114:430-434.
12. Andersson A, Sköld-Larsson K, Hallgren A, Petersson LG, Twetman S. Effect of a dental cream containing amorphous cream phosphate complexes on white spot lesion regression assessed by laser fluorescence. Oral Health Prev Dent 2007;5:229-233.
13. Ekstrand KR, Martignon S, Ricketts DJ, Qvist V. Detection and activity assessment of primary coronal caries lesions: a methodologic study. Oper Dent 2007;32:225-235.
14. Ismail AI, Sohn W, Tellez M, Amaya A, Sen A, Hasson H et al. The International Caries Detection and Assessment System (ICDAS): an integrated system for measuring dental caries. Community Dent Oral Epidemiol 2007;35:170-178.
15. Baeshen HA, Kjellberg H, Lingström P, Birkhed D. Uptake and release of fluoride from fluoride-impregnated chewing sticks (miswaks) in vitro and in vivo. Caries Res 2008;42:363-368.
16. Baeshen H, Birkhed D. Release of fluoride from fresh and old NaF-impregnated chewing sticks (Miswaks) in vitro and oral retention in vivo. Oral Health Prev Dent 2010;In Press.
17. Baeshen H, Kjellberg H, Birkhed D. Oral fluoride retention in orthodontic patients with and without fixed appliances after using different fluoridated home-care products Acta Odontol Scand 2009;In Press.
18. Nordström A, Birkhed D. Fluoride retention in proximal plaque and saliva using two NaF dentifrices containing 5,000 and 1,450 ppm F with and without water rinsing. Caries Res 2009;43:64-69.
19. Rodrigues JA, Hug I, Diniz MB, Lussi A. Performance of fluorescence methods, radiographic examination and ICDAS II on occlusal surfaces in vitro. Caries Res 2008;42:297-304.
20. Bamzahim M, Aljehani A, Shi XQ. Clinical performance of DIAGnodent in the detection of secondary carious lesions. Acta Odontol Scand 2005;63:26-30.
21. Marcusson A, Norevall LI, Persson M. White spot reduction when using glass ionomer cement for bonding in
22. orthodontics: a longitudinal and comparative study. Eur J Orthod 1997;19:233-242.
23. Geiger AM, Gorelick L, Gwinnett AJ, Benson BJ. Reducing white spot lesions in orthodontic populations with fluoride rinsing. Am J Orthod Dentofacial Orthop 1992;101:403-407.
24. Øgaard B, Ten Bosch JJ. Regression of white spot enamel lesions. A new optical method for quantitative longitudinal evaluation in vivo. Am J Orthod Dentofacial Orthop 1994;106:238-242.
25. Al-Khateeb S, Forsberg CM, de Josselin de Jong E, Angmar-Månsson B. A longitudinal laser fluorescence study of white spot lesions in orthodontic patients. Am J Orthod Dentofacial Orthop 1998;113:595-602.

Table I. Scores for the International Caries Detection and Assessment System (ICDAS II).

Score	Meaning
0	**Sound tooth surface**. There should be no evidence of caries (either no or a questionable change in enamel translucency after prolonged air drying (approximately 5 seconds). Surfaces with developmental defects, such as enamel hypoplasias, fluorosis, tooth wear (attrition, abrasion and erosion) and extrinsic or intrinsic stains will be recorded as sound.
1	**First visual change in enamel.** When seen wet, there is no evidence of any change in color that can be attributed to carious activity, but, after prolonged air drying, a carious opacity is visible that is not consistent with the clinical appearance of sound enamel.
2	**Distinct visual change in enamel when viewed wet.** There is a carious opacity or discoloration that is not consistent with the clinical appearance of sound enamel (Note: the lesion is still visible when dry). The lesion is located in close proximity (in touch with or within 1 mm) to the gingival margin.
3	**Localized enamel breakdown due to caries with no visible dentine.** After being dried for 5 seconds, there is carious loss of surface integrity without visible dentine.
4	**Underlying dark shadow from dentine with or without localized enamel breakdown**. This lesion appears as a shadow of discolored dentine visible through the enamel surface beyond the white or brown spot lesion, which may or may not show signs of localized breakdown. This appearance is often seen more easily when the tooth is wet and is a darkening and intrinsic shadow, which may be grey, blue or brown in color.
5	**Distinct cavity with visible dentine**. Cavitation in opaque or discolored enamel exposing the dentine beneath.
6	**Extensive distinct cavity with visible dentine.** Obvious loss of tooth structure, the cavity is both deep and wide and dentine is clearly visible on the walls and at the base. An extensive cavity involves at least half a tooth surface or possibly reaches the pulp.

Table II. Means and standard deviations of the DIAGNOdent and ICDAS II readings for each quadrant in both treatment groups at baseline and at 6 weeks and the changes between the two visits.

Quadrant	DIAGNOdent reading			ICDAS II		
	Baseline	6 weeks	Δ	Baseline	6 weeks	Δ
Test group						
Covered n=19	11.5±6.1	9.2±5.2	-2.3±2.3 ⌐ * * *	2.2±0.7	1.9±0.9	-0.3±0.3 ⌐ * *
Non-covered n=19	13.2±5.6	4.5±2.9	-8.7±3.8 * ⌐ * * * *	2.4±0.8	1.0±0.8	-1.4±0.6 * ⌐ * * * *
Covered – Non-covered			-6.4±3.3 ⌐			-1.2±0.6 ⌐
Control group						
Covered n=18	11.7±7.6	10.1±6.6	-1.5±1.9 * *	1.9±1.0	1.7±1.0	-0.1±0.2 * *
Non-covered n=18	11.5±6.1	9.4±5.3	-2.1±1.9	2.0±0.9	1.7±1.0	-0.3±0.4
Covered – Non-covered			-0.6±2.4 ⌐			-0.2±0.4 ⌐

* * * * $P < 0.0001$

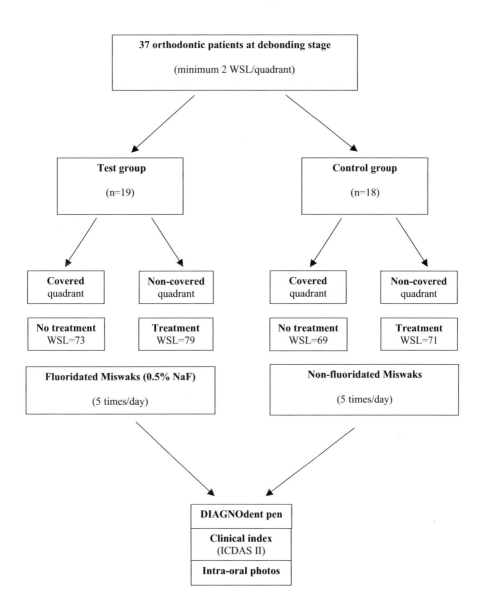

Fig 1.The schematic design of the study.

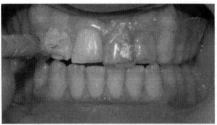

Fig 2. The use of fluoridated Miswaks for cleaning the teeth with a custom-made mouth tray covering half the dentition in the upper jaw. The cleaning was only performed in the non-covered area.

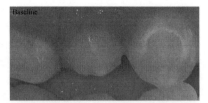

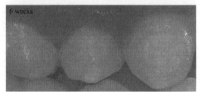

Fig 3. Photos of the non-covered side for one patient in the test group showing the improvement in WSL from baseline to 6 weeks after using F-impregnated Miswaks.

DIAGNOdent Pen

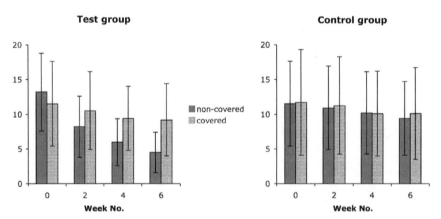

Fig 4. Means and standard deviations of the DIAGNOdent pen readings for covered and non-covered quadrants in both treatment groups at baseline (test group n=19 and control group n=18).

ICDAS II index

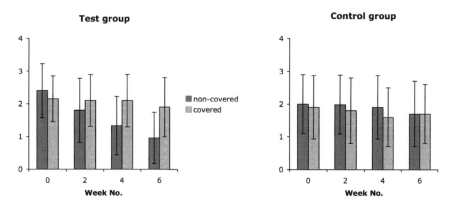

Fig 5. Means and standard deviations of the clinical index (ICDAS II) readings for covered and non-covered quadrants in both treatment groups at baseline (test group n=19 and control group n=18).

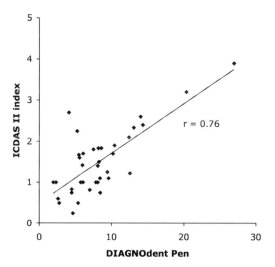

Fig 6. The correlation between the DIAGNOdent readings and the clinical index (ICDAS II) scores at 6 weeks (r=0.76) for all individuals; n=37.